Know Your Fashion

Uncover and Express Your Clothing Style.

By Ally G.

A Show Your Flare Collection

Know Your Fashion: Uncover and Express Your Clothing Style

A Show Your Flare Collection

Identifiers: LCCN 2024918540, ISBN 9798990933538 (PDF), ASIN B0DFX7PK57 (Amazon eBook), ISBN 9798338012307 (Hardcover), ISBN 9798338012154 (Paperback)

The images featured in this book are intended for aesthetic and illustrative purposes only. Remember, everyone has their own unique aesthetic preferences, so feel free to explore your own style ideas without being limited by what you see here.

If you found this book enjoyable, we would love to hear your feedback with a review at the place of purchase. And don't hesitate to visit alloflare.com for a variety of books to further enhance your creative and self-discovery journey.

Table of Contents

Introduction

Purpose of the Book

In a world where first impressions are often formed in mere seconds, the way we present ourselves can shape perceptions and open doors to new opportunities. Fashion is not merely about clothing; it is a dynamic and powerful form of self-expression that allows you to showcase your personality, creativity, and confidence. "Know Your Fashion: Uncover and Express Your Clothing Style" invites you on a transformative journey to discover your unique style and embrace the art of fashion in a way that feels authentic and empowering.

Fashion is a language of its own, speaking volumes about who you are without uttering a single word. From the color of your clothing to the patterns you choose, each detail contributes to the narrative we weave about ourselves. This book seeks to demystify the world of fashion, breaking down the barriers that often make it feel inaccessible or overwhelming. It encourages you to see clothing as a canvas for self-identity, rather than merely a means of covering up.

The purpose of this book is to equip you with the tools, insights, and confidence needed to understand our personal style, navigate the complexities of fashion, and cultivate a wardrobe that genuinely reflects your individuality. Through a blend of practical advice, style tips, and inspirational stories, "Know Your Fashion" aims to help you:

1. Identify Your Style: We will guide you through a process of exploration, where you can discover various fashion influences, styles, and aesthetics. With exercises and prompts, you'll learn to pinpoint what resonates with you, making the journey of self-discovery both enjoyable and enlightening.

2. Build a Versatile Wardrobe: A well-curated wardrobe serves as the foundation of personal style. This book provides strategies for selecting key pieces that are not only stylish but also functional and adaptable for various occasions. You'll learn how to mix and match, layer, and accessorize, ensuring that your wardrobe works for you.

3. Express Yourself: Fashion is a powerful tool for communication. We will delve into how to use clothing as a medium for self-expression, enabling you to articulate who you are without saying a word. Through personal stories and case studies, you'll see how others have embraced their style and gained confidence.

4. Navigate Trends: The world of fashion is ever evolving, with new trends emerging daily. We will help you distinguish between fleeting trends and timeless pieces, empowering you to make informed fashion choices that align with your personal style. You'll learn how to incorporate trends in a way that feels true to you, rather than just following the crowd.

5. Overcome Fashion Challenges: Many people face obstacles when it comes to fashion, whether it's body image issues, lack of inspiration, or confusion about what works for them. This book addresses these challenges head-on, providing practical solutions and encouragement to help you overcome them and celebrate your uniqueness.

6. Cultivate Confidence: Ultimately, the goal of this book is to empower you to feel confident in your clothing choices. We will share tips on how to embrace your body, celebrate your individuality, and adopt a mindset that fosters self-love and acceptance.

By the end of this book, you will not only know your fashion but also feel inspired to express it boldly, confidently, and unapologetically. You will have the tools to navigate the world of fashion with clarity and creativity, allowing you to craft a personal style that is as vibrant and unique as you are. Let this journey begin, and may it lead you to a deeper understanding of yourself and the power of fashion.

The Journey to Personal Style

Embarking on the journey to personal style is much like navigating a rich and diverse landscape. It is an adventure filled with self-discovery, exploration, and creativity. "Know Your Fashion: Uncover and Express Your Clothing Style" is your guidebook for this journey, offering insights and tools to help you understand and articulate your unique fashion identity.

1. Self-Discovery: The first step in this journey is looking inward. Understanding your personality, lifestyle, and preferences is crucial in developing a style that feels truly yours. Through reflective exercises, this book will help you uncover the core elements that influence your fashion choices. Whether you are drawn to bold, vibrant colors or subtle, minimalist designs, recognizing these preferences is the foundation of your personal style.

2. Exploration of Fashion History and Influences: Fashion is ever evolving, influenced by historical events, cultural shifts, and iconic figures. By exploring the rich tapestry of fashion history, you will gain an appreciation for various styles and trends that have shaped the industry. This knowledge not only enriches your understanding but also inspires you to incorporate elements from different eras and cultures into your wardrobe.

3. Practical Guidance: Translating your newfound self-awareness into tangible fashion choices can be challenging. This book provides practical guidance on building a cohesive wardrobe, choosing pieces that complement your body shape, and mixing and matching items to create versatile outfits.

4. Embracing Change and Experimentation: Personal style is not static; it evolves as you do. Embracing change and experimentation is a vital part of this journey. We encourage you to step out of your comfort zone, try new looks, and take fashion risks. This book offers a safe space to explore different styles, providing inspiration and support as you refine your aesthetic.

5. Mindfulness and Sustainability: In today's world, mindful fashion choices are more important than ever. Understanding the impact of your clothing on the environment and society is a crucial aspect of personal style. This book highlights the importance of sustainable fashion practices, from choosing eco-friendly fabrics to supporting ethical brands. By making conscious decisions, you can align your style with your values and contribute to a more sustainable future.

6. Confidence and Authenticity: Ultimately, the goal of this journey is to cultivate confidence and authenticity in your fashion choices. When you dress in a way that feels true to yourself, it radiates confidence and inspires others. This book empowers you to embrace your uniqueness, celebrate your individuality, and express yourself boldly and authentically.

By the end of "Know Your Fashion: Uncover and Express Your Clothing Style," you will not only have a deeper understanding of your personal style but also the confidence to express it with flair and authenticity. This journey is about more than just clothes; it's about celebrating who you are and sharing that with the world through the art of fashion. Let your style journey begin, and may it lead you to a more empowered and vibrant version of yourself.

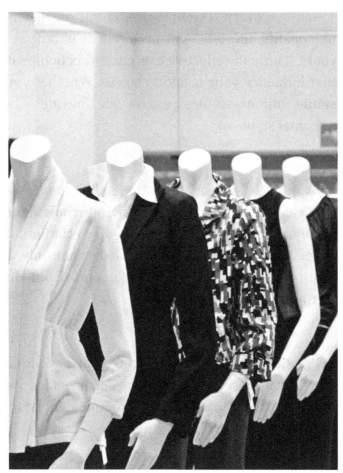

How Fashion Reflects Identity

By understanding the relationship between fashion and identity, we see that fashion is far more than a superficial concern; it is a profound medium through which you communicate your identity to the world. Every choice you make, from the clothes you wear to the accessories you select, is a reflection of your inner selves, and our choices can actually reveal who you are, what you value, and how you see ourselves within the broader context of society.

At its core, fashion serves as a personal billboard. It allows us to project our tastes, beliefs, and moods. Whether through a favorite color, a cherished accessory, or a unique clothing combination, we express our individuality. This book helps you explore how these elements come together to form a cohesive style narrative, empowering you to articulate your identity with clarity and confidence.

In addition, your fashion choices often reflect your cultural background and social affiliations. Traditional attire, for example, can signify heritage and belonging, while contemporary fashion trends can indicate alignment with certain social groups or movements. By understanding the cultural and social dimensions of fashion, you can make more informed choices that resonate with your identity and values.

Furthermore, fashion can also provide us with psychological insights. The psychology of fashion delves into how clothing affects our emotions and perceptions. What you wear can influence your confidence, mood, and even how others perceive you. This book explores the psychological impact of fashion, providing insights into how different styles and colors can enhance your emotional well-being and self-image.

Moreover, in professional settings, fashion plays a crucial role in establishing credibility and authority. The way you dress for work can communicate competence, professionalism, and attention to detail. Fashion also has the power to challenge societal norms and stereotypes. By choosing to wear what truly represents you, you can defy expectations and push boundaries.

As you grow and evolve, so do your fashion choices. Life transitions such as career changes, personal milestones, and shifts in lifestyle can all influence how you dress. This book encourages you to embrace these changes, using fashion as a tool to navigate and celebrate different phases of life. It provides strategies for adapting your wardrobe to new circumstances while staying true to your core identity.

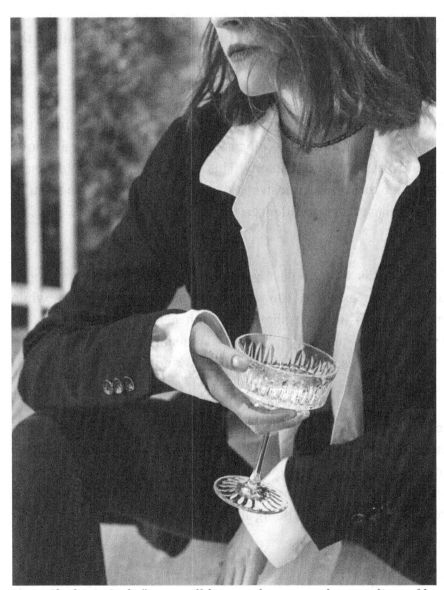

Additionally, in today's world, your fashion choices also reflect your ethical and environmental consciousness. Choosing sustainable and ethically produced clothing speaks to your values and your commitment to a better world. This book offers insights into making fashion choices that are not only stylish but also responsible, allowing you to express your identity with integrity.

By the end of "Know Your Fashion: Uncover and Express Your Clothing Style," you will have a deeper understanding of how fashion reflects and shapes your identity. You will be equipped with the knowledge and confidence to make fashion choices that are authentic, empowering, and aligned with who you are. Embrace the journey of self-expression through fashion, and let your wardrobe become a true reflection of your unique identity.

Overview of Chapters

In Chapter 1: Understanding Fashion Basics, we delve into the fundamental concepts of fashion and personal style. You will learn the difference between fashion — a collective, ever-changing phenomenon — and personal style, which is unique to each individual. We will explore the history and evolution of fashion, tracing significant movements and trends that have shaped the industry. Additionally, we'll identify key fashion terms and concepts, providing you with the vocabulary needed to navigate the fashion world with confidence.

Chapter 2: Discovering Your Personal Style is all about self-discovery and reflection. You will be guided through exercises to reflect on your personal preferences, analyze your lifestyle and needs, and identify fashion inspirations. The culmination of this process will be the creation of a style mood board, a visual representation of your unique fashion identity.

Chapter 3: Building a Versatile Wardrobe you will learn how to curate a wardrobe that is both stylish and functional. This chapter covers essential wardrobe pieces for every style, techniques for mixing basics with statement pieces, and the concept of a capsule wardrobe. You will also find tips on how to adapt your wardrobe seasonally, ensuring that your clothing choices are always appropriate and fashionable.

Color and patterns play a crucial role in fashion. In Chapter 4: Understanding Color and Patterns you will explore the basics of color theory and discover your personal color palette. Learn how to incorporate patterns and textures into your outfits, and how to balance bold and neutral tones to create visually appealing ensembles.

Understanding your body type is essential for creating flattering and comfortable outfits and Chapter 5: Dressing for Your Body Type helps you identify different body shapes and offers tips for finding fits that flatter your figure. You will learn how to emphasize your best features and dress with comfort and confidence.

Accessories can elevate any outfit and Chapter 6: Accessorizing Effectively covers key accessories for every wardrobe, the difference between statement pieces and everyday wear, and how to incorporate jewelry, scarves, and bags into your outfits. You will also learn how to adapt accessories for different seasons, ensuring they complement your overall look.

Shopping smart is about making informed and conscious fashion choices and Chapter 7: Shopping Smart provides tips on budgeting for fashion purchases and finding treasures in thrift and vintage stores. We will also explore how to embrace sustainable and ethical fashion, aligning your purchases with your values.

Chapter 8: Expressing Yourself Through Fashion helps you understand fashion as a form of self-expression and encourages you to try new styles with confidence. You will learn how to balance trends with personal preference and cultivate a unique fashion identity that is true to yourself.

Personal style is an evolving journey and in Chapter 9: Maintaining and Evolving Your Style you will learn how to organize and maintain your wardrobe, update your style with life changes, and stay inspired in fashion. We will explore how to embrace style evolution and growth, ensuring that your fashion choices continue to reflect your evolving self.

This book was created with the purpose of providing you with the necessary knowledge, tools, and confidence to navigate the world of fashion with clarity and creativity, crafting a personal style that is as exceptional and unique as you are.

Definition of Fashion vs. Personal Style

Fashion and personal style are two concepts that, while often intertwined, have distinct meanings and roles in how we present ourselves.

Fashion is the collective term for the prevailing trends and styles in clothing, accessories, and beauty. It is a dynamic and ever-evolving entity, shaped by designers, cultural shifts, technological advancements, and historical events. Fashion is seasonal and cyclical, with trends coming and going as they reflect the zeitgeist of the times. It serves as a mirror of society, capturing the essence of a particular era and translating it into wearable art. Fashion is often showcased through fashion weeks, magazines, and social media, creating a universal language that can be interpreted across cultures.

On the other hand, personal style is deeply individualistic. It is the unique way an individual chooses to express themselves through their clothing and accessories. Unlike fashion, which is transient and influenced by external factors, personal style is enduring and introspective. It is about understanding who you are, what makes you feel confident, and how you want to be perceived by others. Personal style is cultivated over time, often inspired by personal experiences, values, and a sense of identity. It allows individuals to express their creativity and authenticity, going beyond the constraints of current trends.

The interplay between fashion and personal style is what makes the world of clothing so rich and diverse. While fashion provides a plethora of options and inspirations, personal style is about selectively incorporating those elements that resonate with you. It's about curating a wardrobe that balances trendiness with timelessness, ensuring that your clothing is both relevant and reflective of your personality.

To develop a strong sense of personal style, it's important to explore different fashion trends, experiment with various silhouettes and colors, and pay attention to what feels most comfortable and true to yourself. Embracing personal style does not mean disregarding fashion; rather, it means engaging with fashion thoughtfully, using it as a tool to enhance your self-expression.

By understanding the distinction between fashion and personal style, you can cultivate a wardrobe that not only aligns with contemporary trends but also resonates with your personal identity. This balance allows you to remain current while staying true to yourself, creating a harmonious blend of the external and internal aspects of style.

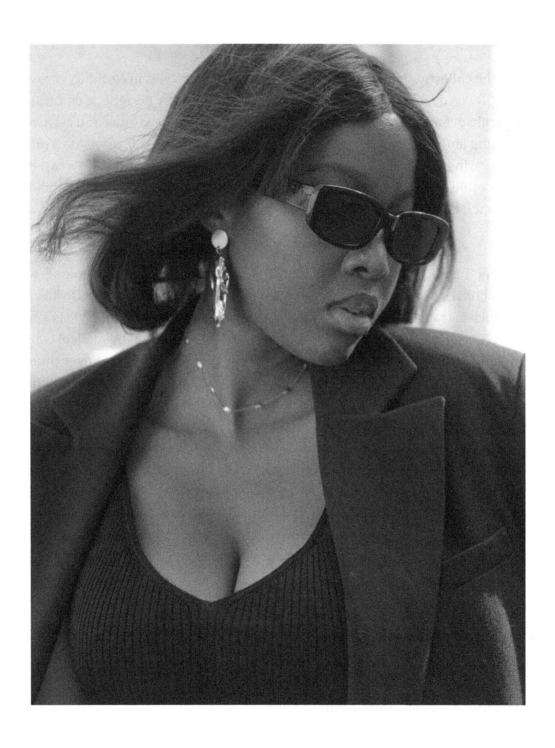

History and Evolution of Fashion

The history and evolution of fashion is a captivating narrative that mirrors the cultural, social, and technological transformations throughout human civilization.

In ancient times, fashion was not just about aesthetics, but also practicality and status. In Egypt, clothing was predominantly made from linen, a lightweight fabric ideal for the region's climate. The color and quality of the linen often indicated one's social status, with the elite donning finely woven and intricately pleated garments. Jewelry played a significant role, symbolizing power and protection.

In ancient Greece, fashion emphasized harmony and proportion. The chiton and himation were popular garments, made from rectangular pieces of fabric draped elegantly around the body. These garments allowed for freedom of movement and were often adorned with decorative borders.

The Middle Ages introduced more structured garments. Clothing became a clear indicator of social hierarchy. The nobility wore elaborate garments made from luxurious fabrics like silk and brocade, while the lower classes wore simpler wool and linen attire. The introduction of the spinning wheel and improvements in weaving techniques led to more varied and intricate textiles.

Sumptuary laws emerged, dictating what individuals could wear, aiming to maintain class distinctions. This period also saw the development of tailoring, leading to more fitted and individualized clothing.

The Renaissance was a period of rebirth in art and culture, which was vividly reflected in fashion. Clothing became more expressive and detailed, with an emphasis on opulence. The use of rich fabrics such as velvet and silk, along with elaborate embroidery and lace, became widespread. Fashion became an important aspect of court life, with rulers using it as a means to display power and wealth.

The Renaissance also saw the rise of fashion as an industry, with the establishment of workshops and the emergence of fashion designers who began to gain recognition for their work.

The 18th century was marked by extravagance, especially in France under the reign of Louis XIV, where fashion was a key element of court culture. The elaborate gowns, powdered wigs, and intricate accessories of this era reflected the opulence and hierarchical nature of society.

The 19th century brought about major changes due to the Industrial Revolution. The invention of the sewing machine and advances in textile production made clothing more affordable and accessible. This democratization of fashion allowed for broader participation in fashion trends, paving the way for the rise of department stores and ready-to-wear garments.

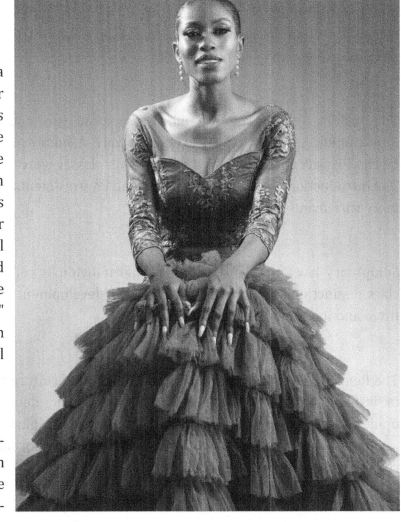

The 20th century was a groundbreaking period for fashion. The early decades saw the rise of haute couture, with designers like Coco Chanel and Christian Dior redefining women's fashion with their innovative designs. Chanel introduced a more relaxed and practical style, while Dior's "New Look" celebrated femininity with its cinched waists and full skirts.

Moving on to the mid-century, the fashion industry expanded with the introduction of ready-to-wear collections, making fashion more accessible. The 1960s and 70s were characterized by youth-driven fashion movements, with styles reflecting social and political changes. The 1980s embraced bold colors and extravagant styles, symbolizing the economic boom and cultural excesses of the era.

In the 21st century, fashion continues to evolve rapidly, driven by globalization and digital advancements. Sustainability has become a critical focus, with designers and brands prioritizing eco-friendly materials and ethical production practices. The rise of fast fashion has made trends more accessible but also raised concerns about environmental impacts.

Social media has revolutionized how fashion is consumed and shared, creating a more interactive and immediate fashion landscape. Influencers and digital platforms now play a significant role in shaping trends and consumer preferences.

The evolution of fashion is a reflection of human creativity, cultural exchange, and technological progress. It not only showcases changes in style but also mirrors the shifting values and aspirations of society. Understanding this rich history enhances our appreciation for fashion as both an art form and a powerful medium of self-expression, highlighting its enduring impact on the world.

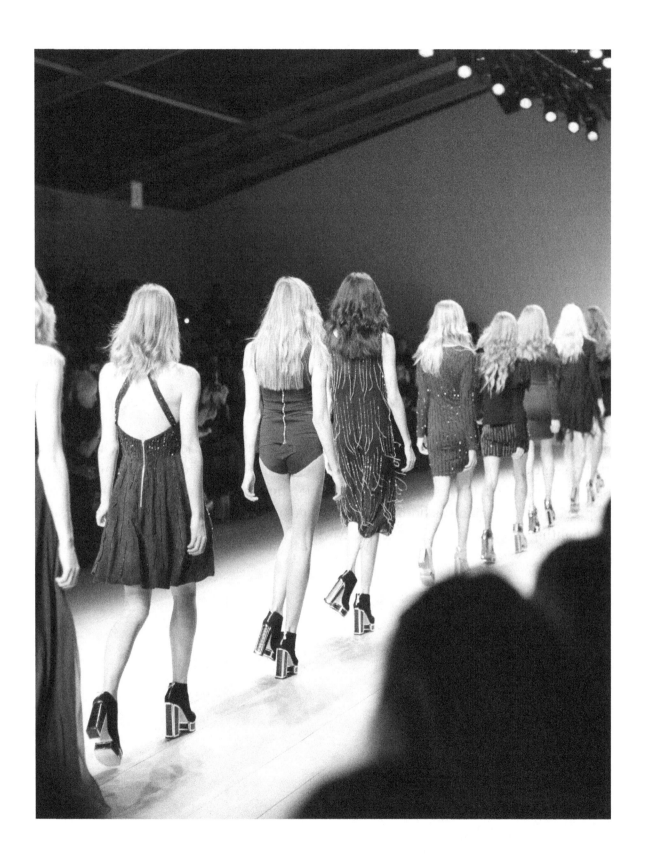

Identifying Key Fashion Terms and Concepts

Navigating the intricate world of fashion requires familiarity with a variety of terms and concepts that help define styles, trends, and the industry itself. Here's a quick guide to some essential fashion terminology:

A

- Accessory: An item added to an outfit to enhance its overall look, such as jewelry, bags, hats, and scarves.

- A-line: A silhouette that is fitted at the top and flares out towards the hem, resembling the shape of the letter "A."

- Avant-garde: Fashion that is innovative, experimental, or ahead of its time, often challenging traditional norms.

B

- Bespoke: Custom-made clothing, tailored specifically to an individual's measurements and preferences.

- Bohemian: A style characterized by relaxed, artistic, and often vintage-inspired clothing, often with ethnic or gypsy influences.

- Brocade: A rich fabric, typically made with silk, featuring raised patterns, often used in formal wear.

C

- Chic: A term used to describe a stylish, fashionable, and sophisticated appearance.

- Capsule wardrobe: A small collection of versatile clothing pieces that can be mixed and matched to create multiple outfits.

- Couture: High-end fashion design that is custom-fitted and made from high-quality, expensive fabrics.

D

- Drape: The way fabric hangs and falls on the body, which can affect the overall silhouette of a garment.

- Denim: A sturdy cotton twill fabric, often associated with jeans and casual wear.

- Duster: A long, lightweight coat that is typically open at the front, often worn for layering.

E

- Embellishment: Decorative details added to garments, such as beads, sequins, or embroidery.

- Ethereal: A style that is light, delicate, and almost otherworldly in appearance.

- Empire waist: A dress design where the waistline is raised, sitting just below the bust, creating a flowing skirt.

F

- Fast fashion: Inexpensive clothing produced rapidly by mass-market retailers in response to the latest trends.

- Fit: The way a garment conforms to the body, including tightness and looseness.

- Floral print: A pattern featuring flowers, commonly used in dresses and casual wear.

G

- Glamour: A style that emphasizes elegance and allure, often associated with high fashion and luxury.

- Gingham: A checked pattern of alternating colored squares, often used in casual clothing.

- Gore: A triangular or trapezoidal piece of fabric inserted into a garment to add fullness or shape.

H

- Haute couture: High fashion that is made-to-order for specific clients, featuring the highest quality materials and craftsmanship.

- Harem pants: Loose-fitting trousers that are snug at the ankles and often have a dropped crotch.

- Hemline: The bottom edge of a garment, which can vary in length.

I

- Inseam: The measurement of the inner seam of pants, indicating the length from the crotch to the hem.

- Issey Miyake: A renowned Japanese fashion designer known for his innovative pleating techniques and textile designs.

- Illusion neckline: A sheer fabric at the neckline creating the appearance of a floating collar or décolletage.

J

- Jumpsuit: A one-piece garment that combines a top and pants, often used for both casual and formal wear.

- Jersey: A stretchable fabric, typically made from cotton or synthetic fibers, commonly used in t-shirts and casual wear.

- Jacket: A lightweight, outer garment that typically has sleeves and is worn over other clothing.

K

- Kimono: A traditional Japanese garment characterized by long sleeves and a wrap-around design.

- Knitwear: Clothing made from knitted fabric, such as sweaters and cardigans.

- Knee-length: Referring to garments that end at or near the knees.

L

- Linen: A lightweight, breathable fabric made from flax, known for its crisp texture and natural luster.

- Layering: The practice of wearing multiple clothing items on top of one another for style or warmth.

- Lapel: The folded part of a collar that is sewn onto the garment, often found on jackets and coats.

M

- Merino wool: A type of fine wool obtained from merino sheep, known for its softness and warmth.

- Midi: A length that falls between the knee and ankle, often used to describe skirts and dresses.

- Monochrome: An outfit composed of different shades of a single color.

N

- Neckline: The top edge of a garment that surrounds the neck, which can come in various styles (e.g., V-neck, crew neck).

- Nautical: A style inspired by maritime themes, often featuring stripes, anchors, and colors like navy blue and white.

- Nude: A color that closely resembles the skin tone, often used in footwear and undergarments to create a seamless look.

O

- Off-the-shoulder: A style where the garment sits below the shoulders, exposing the collarbone and shoulders.

- Oversized: A fit that is intentionally larger than standard sizes, often for a relaxed or casual look.

- Oxford shirt: A classic button-up shirt made from Oxford cloth, known for its durability and versatility.

P

- Pleats: Folds in fabric that are sewn into place, adding texture and volume to garments like skirts and trousers.

- Peplum: A short, gathered, or pleated strip of fabric at the waist of a garment, often used to create a flared effect.

- Pattern: A repeated decorative design printed or woven into fabric.

Q

- Quilted: Fabric that has been stitched together in a pattern to create a padded effect, often used in jackets and bags.

- Quirk: A unique or unconventional detail in a garment or accessory that adds character or individuality.

R

- Ready-to-wear: Clothing that is mass-produced and sold in standard sizes, as opposed to custom-made garments.

- Romper: A one-piece garment that combines a top and shorts, typically casual and comfortable.

- Ruching: A technique where fabric is gathered or pleated to create a textured effect, often used in dresses and skirts.

S

- Silhouette: The overall shape and outline of a garment, which can convey different styles and aesthetics.

- Streetwear: A casual fashion style characterized by urban influences, often featuring graphic tees, hoodies, and sneakers.

- Sustainable fashion: Clothing designed with environmentally friendly practices, focusing on ethical production and materials.

T

- Tailoring: The art of fitting and adjusting garments to enhance fit and style, often associated with bespoke clothing.

- Tulle: A lightweight, sheer fabric often used in skirts and veils, known for its airy quality.

- Trench coat: A long, waterproof coat with a belted waist and typically double-breasted, originally designed for military use.

U

- Upcycling: The process of repurposing old or discarded clothing into new, higher-quality items.

- Unisex: Clothing designed to be worn by any gender, often characterized by neutral styles and fits.

V

- Vogue: A term used to describe the prevailing fashion style or trend, also the name of a famous fashion magazine.

- Vintage: Clothing that is at least 20 years old, often sought after for its unique style and historical significance.

- V-neck: A neckline style shaped like the letter "V," which can be flattering and elongating.

W

- Wardrobe: A collection of clothing and accessories that a person owns.

- Wrap dress: A dress that wraps around the body and ties at the waist, known for its flattering fit on various body types.

- Wool: A natural fiber obtained from sheep, known for its warmth and versatility in clothing.

X

- X-ray fashion: A style that incorporates sheer or transparent fabrics, revealing the layers beneath without full exposure.

- X-factor: A term used in fashion to describe a unique quality or characteristic that makes a look stand out.

Y

- Yoke: A fitted piece of fabric that connects the bodice of a garment to the skirt or lower part, often found in shirts and dresses.

- Youth culture: Fashion influenced by the styles and trends popular among younger generations, often characterized by casual and edgy designs.

Z

- Zipper: A fastening device used in clothing, bags, and accessories, consisting of two strips of fabric with interlocking metal or plastic teeth.

- Zodiac fashion: Styles that are inspired by astrological signs, often incorporating colors and symbols associated with each sign.

Familiarizing yourself with these key fashion terms and concepts deepens your understanding and appreciation of the fashion industry. This knowledge empowers you to make informed choices about your personal style and engage more deeply with fashion as both a consumer and an enthusiast, navigating trends with confidence and creativity.

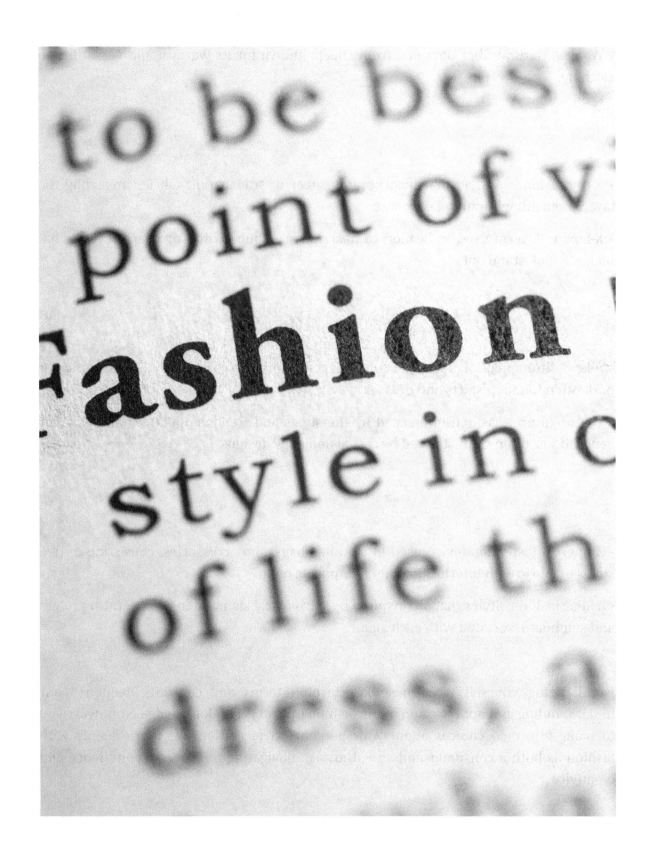

to be best
point of vi
Fashion
style in c
of life th
dress, a

Chapter 2:

Discovering Your

Personal Style

Reflecting on Personal Preferences

Embarking on the journey to discover your personal style is an exciting exploration of self-expression and individuality. This chapter invites you to delve deeply into your personal preferences, the foundation upon which your unique style is built. By reflecting on what truly resonates with you, you can craft a wardrobe that not only reflects your personality but also enhances your confidence and comfort.

Understanding Your Likes and Dislikes

Begin by exploring the colors, patterns, and textures that naturally draw your interest. Take note of the hues that excite you or bring you peace. Are you captivated by bold, vibrant colors, or do you prefer the serenity of soft, muted tones? Consider the patterns that appeal to you—are you drawn to intricate designs, or do you favor simple, clean lines? Understanding these preferences is crucial in forming a clearer picture of your style.

Lifestyle and Practicality

Your lifestyle plays a significant role in shaping your personal style. Reflect on your daily routine and the environments you frequent. Are you often in professional settings, requiring a more formal wardrobe, or do you spend more time in casual, relaxed spaces? Perhaps your lifestyle demands versatility, allowing for a seamless transition between different settings. Understanding how your wardrobe needs to function in your life will guide you in making choices that are both stylish and practical.

Emotional Connection

Style is not just about aesthetics; it's also about how clothing makes you feel. Reflect on the emotions that different styles evoke within you. Do certain outfits make you feel confident and empowered, while others bring comfort and relaxation? Consider the pieces that hold sentimental value or boost your mood. Identifying these emotional connections will guide you in choosing pieces that resonate with your authentic self, making your wardrobe a source of joy and empowerment.

Inspiration and Aspiration

Draw inspiration from a variety of sources, such as fashion magazines, social media, art, nature, and even the people around you. What styles do you admire, and why? Take note of the elements that captivate you. While it's important to stay true to yourself, allowing yourself to be inspired by others can open up new possibilities and help refine your style. Aspiration plays a role too—consider the image you wish to project and how your style can align with your personal and professional goals.

Creating a Style Vision Board

One effective way to bring your reflections to life is by creating a style vision board. Gather images, fabrics, and color swatches that resonate with you. This visual representation will serve as a guide and reminder of the personal preferences that define your style. It's a creative exercise that not only clarifies your vision but also inspires new ideas and combinations you may not have considered before.

Experimentation and Evolution

Remember that discovering your personal style is an ongoing journey. Allow yourself the freedom to experiment and evolve. Try new combinations, step out of your comfort zone, and embrace change. Your preferences may shift over time, and that's perfectly natural. By staying open to new experiences and ideas, you'll find that your style will continue to grow and adapt, reflecting the person you are becoming.

By taking the time to reflect on your personal preferences, you lay a strong foundation for discovering a style that is uniquely yours. Embrace this process of self-discovery with an open mind and a joyful heart. Let your personal style be a true reflection of who you are—a celebration of your individuality and a testament to your journey.

Analyzing Your Lifestyle and Needs

Understanding your lifestyle and daily needs is a crucial step in curating a wardrobe that is both functional and reflective of your personal style. By thoughtfully analyzing how you spend your time and what your day-to-day activities entail, you can ensure your clothing choices enhance your life, rather than complicate it.

Daily Activities and Environment

Begin by charting out your typical daily activities. Are you working in a traditional office setting, or does your routine involve more dynamic environments like a bustling city or a home office? Each scenario demands different attire. For example, a corporate setting might require tailored suits and formal wear, while a more relaxed or creative environment might allow for casual or eclectic styles. Understanding where you spend most of your time will help you select clothing that integrates seamlessly into your daily routine.

Functional Requirements

Consider the functional aspects of your wardrobe. Do you need pieces that allow for a lot of movement, such as walking or commuting by bike? Or perhaps your lifestyle requires you to transition from professional meetings to social gatherings with ease. Versatility becomes key here, with items that can adapt to different settings and activities. Think about incorporating multi-functional pieces like blazers that can be dressed up or down, or comfortable footwear that still looks polished.

Climate and Seasonality

The climate you live in plays a pivotal role in shaping your wardrobe needs. Analyze the weather patterns in your area to determine the types of clothing required throughout the year. If you live in a region with distinct seasons, it's important to build a wardrobe that includes warm layers for winter, breathable fabrics for summer, and transitional pieces for the in-between months. For more consistent climates, focus on materials that offer comfort and durability year-round, such as lightweight cottons or merino wool.

Personal and Professional Balance

Reflect on the balance between your personal and professional life. Do you require a clear distinction between work attire and casual wear, or does your lifestyle allow for more fluidity between the two? This balance will influence how you allocate resources when building your wardrobe. For example, if your work environment is formal, investing in high-quality suits or dresses may be essential, whereas a more casual workplace might allow for a greater focus on versatile, everyday pieces.

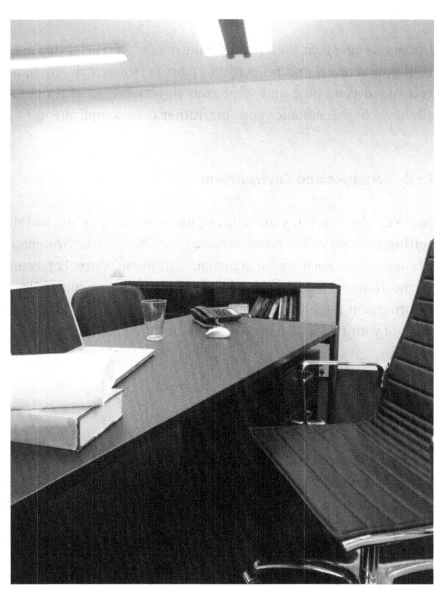

Special Occasions and Hobbies

In addition to day-to-day needs, consider the special occasions and hobbies that are a part of your life. Whether it's attending formal events, engaging in outdoor activities, going to the gym, or pursuing artistic endeavors, having a few key pieces tailored to these activities will enrich your wardrobe. Assess the frequency of these events and prioritize accordingly, ensuring that you're prepared for any occasion without feeling overwhelmed.

Budget Considerations

Analyzing your lifestyle also involves understanding your budget and how it aligns with your clothing needs. Determine where to invest in high-quality staples that will stand the test of time, and where you can opt for more affordable, trend-focused items that refresh your wardrobe. A well-thought-out budget ensures that your wardrobe remains both stylish and sustainable over time, allowing you to make mindful purchases that support your lifestyle.

Sustainability and Ethical Considerations

Finally, consider the values that are important to you, such as sustainability and ethical fashion. Reflect on how these values can be incorporated into your wardrobe choices. Opting for sustainable materials, supporting ethical brands, and choosing quality over quantity are ways to ensure your wardrobe aligns with your principles, adding another layer of satisfaction to your style journey.

By thoroughly analyzing your lifestyle and needs, you can create a wardrobe that not only reflects your personal style but also enhances your daily life. This thoughtful approach leads to a more cohesive, functional, and fulfilling wardrobe, empowering you to move through life with confidence and ease.

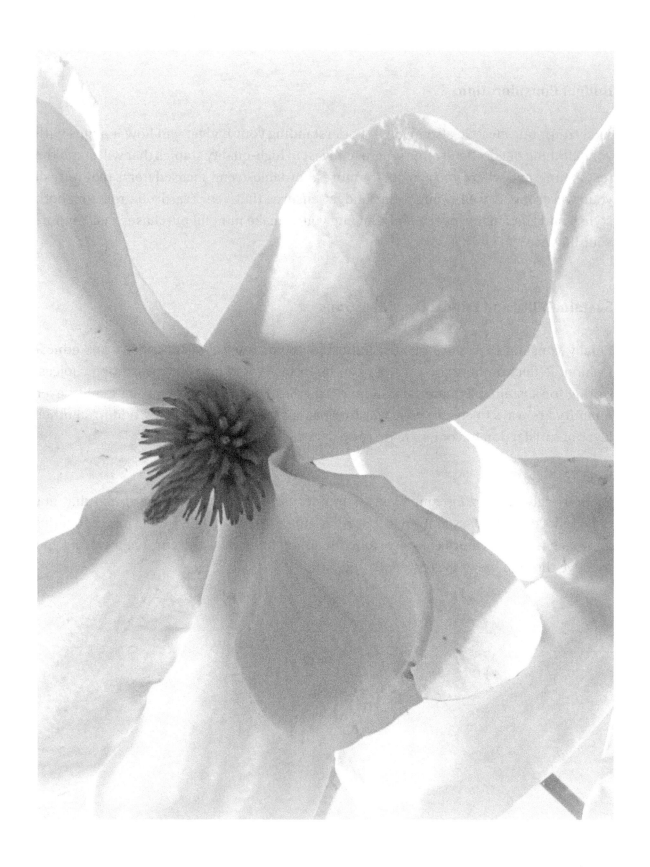

Identifying Fashion Inspirations

Embarking on the journey to discover your personal style is enriched by tapping into the diverse influences and inspirations around you. Identifying fashion inspirations is a crucial step in crafting a style that feels both authentic and unique. By exploring various sources of inspiration, you can develop a style that truly resonates with your personality and aspirations.

Exploring Diverse Sources

Begin by exploring a wide array of sources for fashion inspiration. Fashion magazines, blogs, and social media platforms like Instagram and Pinterest offer a wealth of ideas. These platforms allow you to explore endless styles, from avant-garde to classic, and can help you identify patterns in what appeals to you. Pay attention to designers, influencers, or celebrities whose style you admire. Are there particular elements—such as color palettes, silhouettes, or accessories—that consistently catch your eye? These insights can be instrumental in shaping your own preferences.

Cultural and Historical Influences

Consider the impact of cultural and historical influences on your style. Different eras and cultures offer unique aesthetics that can add depth and character to your wardrobe. Are you drawn to the elegance of the 1920s, the rebellious spirit of the 1960s, or the boldness of the 1980s? Perhaps elements of Japanese minimalism or African prints resonate with you. These influences can help you incorporate meaningful elements into your wardrobe, adding both depth and personal significance.

Art and Nature

Art and nature are profound sources of inspiration that can influence your fashion choices in unique ways. The colors, shapes, and textures found in art can translate beautifully into clothing and accessories. Consider how the fluid lines of a painting or the vibrant hues of a sculpture might inspire your fashion choices. Similarly, nature's palette and patterns can inspire everything from the prints you choose to the colors you wear.

The rich greens of a forest or the soft pastels of a sunset might influence your wardrobe's color scheme, bringing a unique touch to your style.

Personal Icons and Role Models

Reflect on the personal icons and role models who inspire you. These could be figures from your own life, such as family members, mentors, or friends whose style you admire. Consider what it is about their style that appeals to you. Is it their confidence, their ability to mix and match pieces, or their adherence to timeless classics? Identifying these traits can help you emulate aspects of their style while making it your own. Remember, the goal is to draw inspiration from their essence, not to replicate their style exactly.

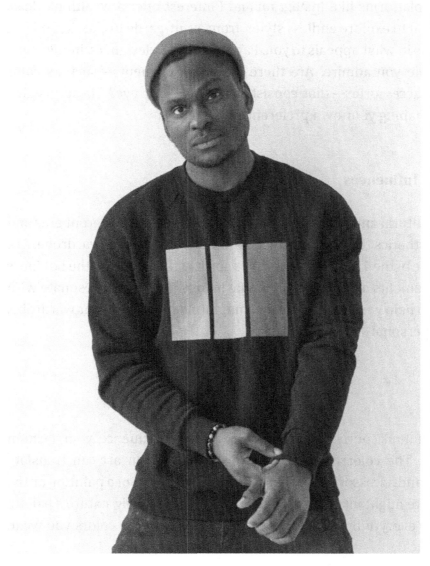

Fashion Shows and Street Style

Fashion shows and street style offer dynamic and ever-evolving sources of inspiration. Watching runway shows can expose you to the latest trends and innovative styling ideas, while street style captures real-world fashion in diverse settings. While runway styles might be more extravagant, they can inspire you to experiment with new silhouettes, colors, and accessories in ways that suit your lifestyle. Street style, on the other hand, often provides practical ideas for incorporating trends into everyday wear.

Creating an Inspiration Board

To organize your inspirations, consider creating an inspiration board. Compile images, fabric swatches, and sketches that resonate with you. This visual representation serves as a tangible collection of your influences, helping you to identify common themes and ideas. Over time, this board can evolve, reflecting your growing and changing sense of style. It can also serve as a creative outlet, allowing you to play with combinations and concepts before trying them out in real life.

Adapting and Personalizing Inspirations

Finally, remember that inspiration is a starting point, not a destination. Adapt and personalize what you admire to fit your own tastes and lifestyle. Mix different elements to create a look that feels uniquely yours. The goal is not to replicate someone else's style, but to develop a wardrobe that reflects your individuality and makes you feel confident. Allow your inspirations to guide you, but always stay true to yourself.

By identifying and embracing your fashion inspirations, you empower yourself to craft a personal style that is both expressive and authentic. Let these inspirations guide you on your style journey, helping you to make thoughtful choices that celebrate who you are.

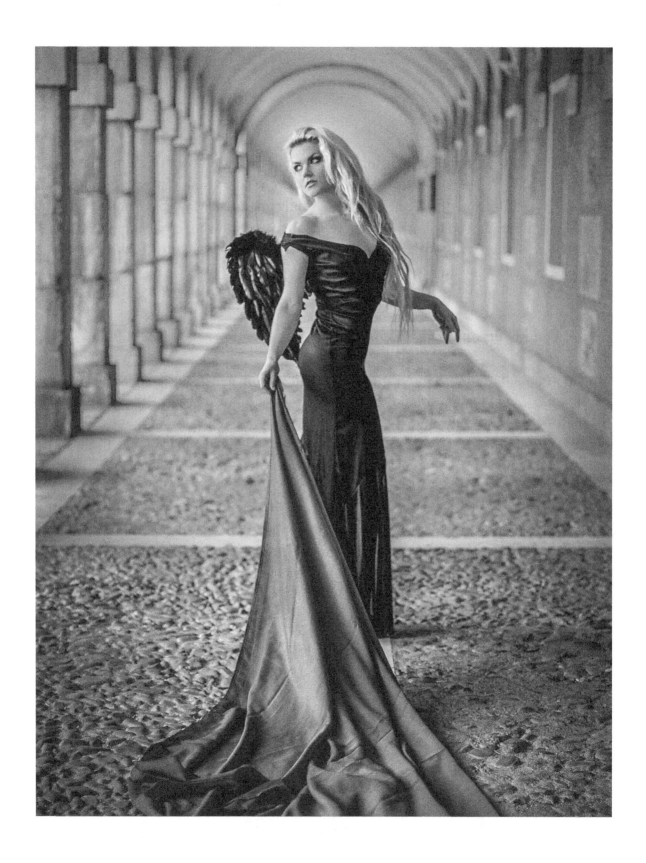

Creating a Style Mood Board

A style mood board is a dynamic and creative tool that helps you visualize and refine your personal style. It serves as a canvas for gathering inspiration, exploring ideas, and seeing how different elements harmonize. By creating a mood board, you can clarify your style vision, make more intentional fashion choices, and embark on a journey of self-expression.

Gathering Inspiration

Begin by collecting a wide variety of images that resonate with you. These might include photos from fashion magazines, designer lookbooks, or snapshots of street style. Consider incorporating images from art, architecture, and nature—anything that captures your aesthetic sensibilities. The goal is to gather a rich tapestry of inspiration that reflects your tastes and aspirations.

Defining Themes and Concepts

As you gather images, start identifying recurring themes or concepts. Are there specific colors, patterns, or textures that frequently appear? Do certain styles or silhouettes stand out to you? Look for connections—such as a preference for minimalist lines or vibrant, eclectic patterns—that can guide your style choices. These themes will help you understand your preferences and refine your personal style vision.

Organizing Your Board

Once you have a collection of images, it's time to organize them on your mood board. You can create a physical board using materials like corkboard, poster board, or scrapbooks, or opt for a digital version using platforms like Pinterest, Canva, or Milanote. Arrange your images in a way that feels cohesive and balanced. Consider creating sections for different aspects of your style, such as casual wear, professional attire, and evening looks. This organization allows you to see how various elements interact and complement one another.

Adding Texture and Color

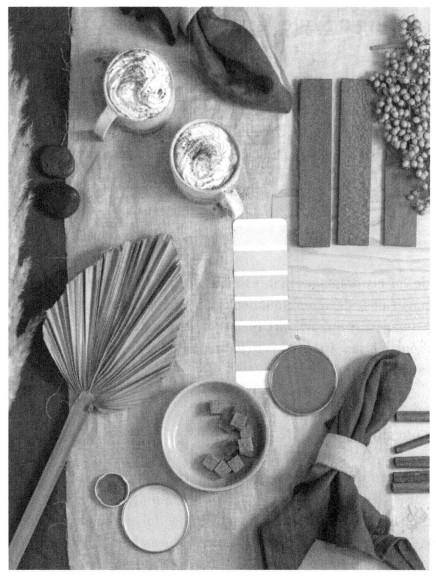

Enhance your mood board by incorporating texture and color swatches. Add fabric samples, paint chips, or even small objects like buttons or beads that reflect the tactile elements of your style. This not only adds depth to your board but also helps you visualize how different materials and colors work together. Consider the emotional responses these textures and colors evoke, and how they align with the image you wish to project.

Reflecting on Your Choices

Take time to reflect on your completed mood board. What does it reveal about your personal style? Are there any surprising insights or new directions you hadn't considered before? Use this reflection to refine your board, adding or removing elements as needed. Your mood board should be a living document that evolves with you, capturing shifts in your style preferences and lifestyle changes over time.

Using Your Mood Board as a Guide

With your mood board in place, use it as a guide for building and curating your wardrobe. Refer to it when shopping for new pieces or assembling outfits. It will serve as a visual reminder of your style goals, helping you make cohesive and confident fashion decisions. Whether you're exploring a new trend or investing in timeless staples, your mood board will keep you aligned with your unique aesthetic.

Evolving Your Mood Board

Remember, your style mood board is not static. As your tastes, lifestyle, and inspirations evolve, update your board to reflect these changes. Regularly revisiting and revising your mood board ensures that your style remains fresh and aligned with your current self. Embrace this ongoing process as a means of self-discovery and creative expression, allowing your style to grow alongside you.

By creating and continually evolving a style mood board, you gain a deeper understanding of your personal style and a powerful tool for expressing it. Embrace this creative process to craft a wardrobe that truly resonates with your unique identity and enhances your confidence and self-expression.

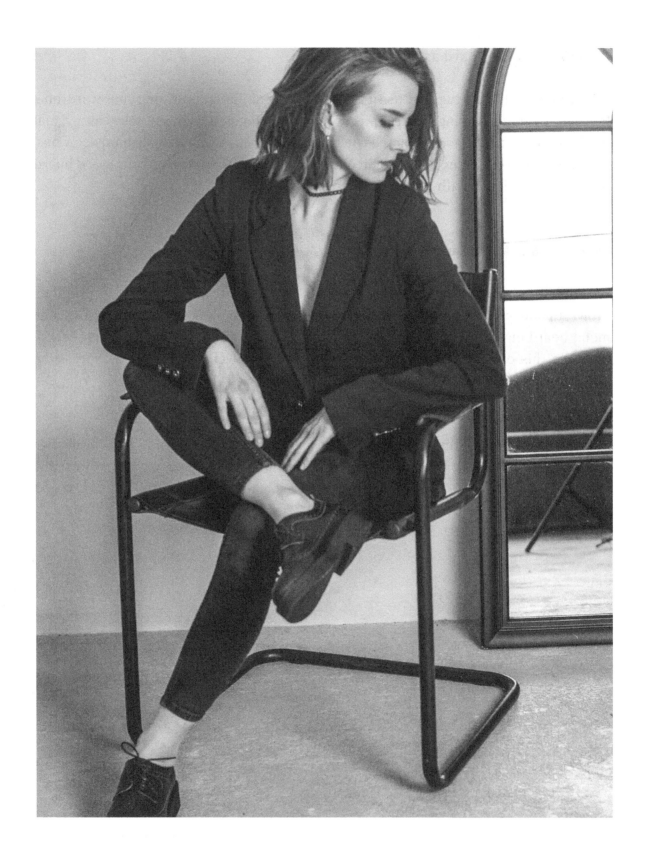

Chapter 3:

Building a Versatile

Wardrobe

Essential Wardrobe Pieces for Every Style

Building a versatile wardrobe is the cornerstone of achieving effortless style and confidence. It's about curating a collection of clothing that allows for endless mixing and matching, adapting to various occasions, seasons, and personal tastes. This chapter explores the essential wardrobe pieces that create a strong foundation, ensuring you're prepared for any situation with grace and flair.

The Classic White Shirt

A crisp white shirt is unparalleled in its versatility. It serves as a blank canvas, allowing for both minimalist and bold fashion statements. Pair it with tailored trousers for a polished office look or wear it casually with jeans and sneakers. Opt for high-quality fabric and a flattering fit to ensure longevity and comfort.

The Little Black Dress

The little black dress (LBD) is a timeless staple, celebrated for its adaptability. Whether attending a cocktail party or a business dinner, the LBD can be your go-to outfit. Enhance its elegance with statement jewelry and heels, or keep it understated with a cardigan and ballet flats. The key is to choose a style that complements your body shape and suits multiple occasions.

A Well-Fitted Blazer

A tailored blazer can transform any outfit, adding a touch of sophistication. It's perfect for layering over a dress or pairing with jeans and a t-shirt for a smart-casual look. Consider investing in a blazer in a neutral color like black, navy, or gray, which can seamlessly integrate into various ensembles.

Quality Denim Jeans

Denim jeans are a quintessential part of any wardrobe, offering comfort and style. A well-fitted pair of jeans can transition effortlessly from day to night. Whether you prefer skinny, straight-leg, or bootcut, choose a style that suits your body and lifestyle. A dark wash is particularly versatile, suitable for both casual and semi-formal settings.

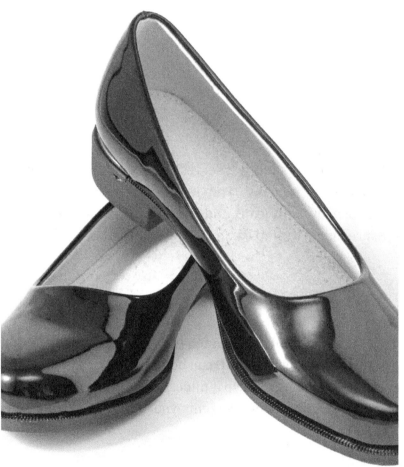

Comfortable Flats and Versatile Heels

Shoes play a critical role in defining an outfit's tone. Comfortable flats are essential for everyday activities, providing ease without sacrificing style. Look for classic ballet flats or loafers in neutral tones. For special occasions, a pair of versatile heels can add elegance and lengthen your silhouette. Choose a style that complements most of your wardrobe and offers comfort for extended wear.

The Neutral Sweater

A neutral-colored sweater is a cozy and stylish addition to any wardrobe. It's perfect for layering, providing warmth and texture without overwhelming an outfit. Opt for quality materials like cashmere or wool for a luxurious feel and durability. Pair it with jeans for a relaxed look or layer it over a dress for added dimension.

Tailored Trousers

Tailored trousers in a neutral shade are indispensable for both work and casual settings. They offer a polished appearance and can be dressed up with a blouse and blazer or dressed down with a simple t-shirt. Look for trousers with a flattering cut and high-quality fabric to ensure comfort and longevity.

The Timeless Trench Coat

A trench coat is a classic outerwear piece that combines practicality with style. Ideal for transitional weather, it adds sophistication to any outfit. Choose a neutral color and a length that suits your height and body type. The trench coat's timeless appeal ensures it remains a staple in your wardrobe for years to come.

Versatile Accessories

Accessories are the finishing touches to any outfit, allowing for personalization and creativity. Scarves, belts, and statement jewelry can transform a simple ensemble into something remarkable. Invest in pieces that reflect your personality and can be easily integrated with your wardrobe. A colorful scarf or bold necklace can add interest and vibrancy to neutral clothing.

A Reliable Handbag

A high-quality handbag in a neutral color is a functional and fashionable addition to your wardrobe. It should be spacious enough to carry your essentials while maintaining a sleek appearance. Consider the bag's material and craftsmanship, as a well-made handbag can elevate any outfit and serve you well for years.

As you can see, by focusing on these essential pieces, you can build a wardrobe that is both versatile and reflective of your personal style. The key is to choose items that complement each other, offer comfort, and adapt to various occasions. With the right foundation, you can effortlessly create endless outfit combinations that express your unique fashion sense and meet your lifestyle needs.

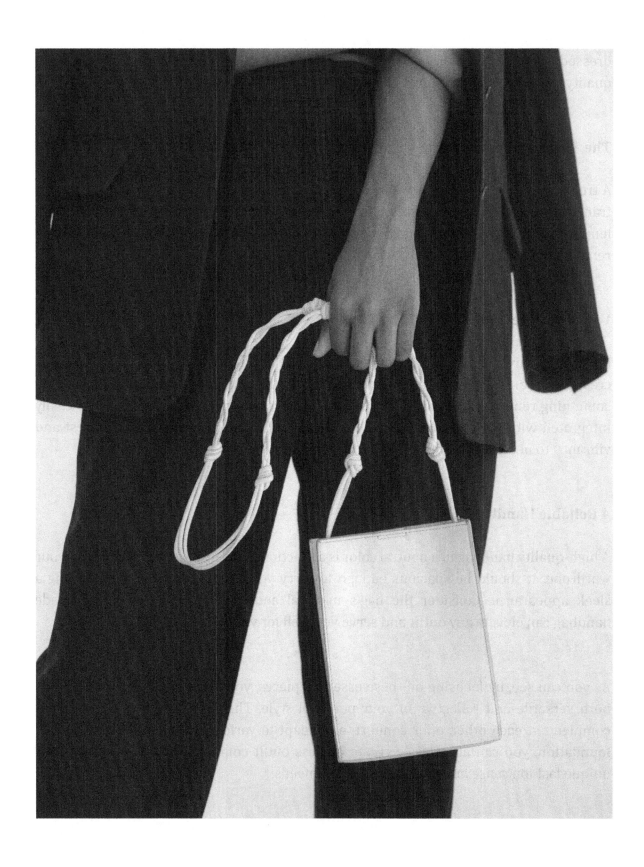

Mixing Basics with Statement Pieces

Now that we have covered some essential basic pieces, we can now bring more personality to your looks by adding statement pieces. Integrating basics with statement pieces is an art that elevates your wardrobe, allowing personal expression while maintaining versatility. Here's a detailed guide on mastering this balance:

Understanding the Basics

Basics are the foundational elements of your wardrobe. These include classic items such as plain t-shirts, neutral sweaters, tailored trousers, and simple jeans. They are versatile, timeless, and form the backbone of any outfit, providing a blank canvas that can be styled in myriad ways.

Versatility:

Basics are adaptable, easily transitioning from day to night or casual to formal with the addition of different accessories or outerwear.

Timeless Appeal:

These pieces never go out of style, making them a wise investment for the long term.

Neutral Palette:

Often in neutral tones like black, white, gray, and beige, basics can be mixed and matched effortlessly.

Introducing Statement Pieces

Statement pieces are bold, eye-catching items that express individuality and fashion-forward thinking. These can include vibrant patterns, unique cuts, or standout accessories like elaborate jewelry or artistic shoes.

Vibrancy and Color:

Bright colors or unusual patterns draw attention and add energy to an outfit.

Unique Design:

Items with unique silhouettes or intricate details become focal points of your ensemble.

Expressive Accessories:

Statement jewelry, scarves, or hats can add flair and personality to otherwise simple outfits.

Balancing the Two

Focus on One Statement Piece:

Choose one item to be the focal point and keep the rest of your outfit simple. This prevents the look from becoming overwhelming. For example, wear a bold patterned skirt with a plain top.

Use Accessories to Elevate Basics:

Transform a basic outfit with statement accessories. A simple white shirt paired with a colorful necklace or bold handbag creates interest and depth, allowing you to experiment with different looks without committing to a full statement outfit.

Mix Textures and Fabrics:

Combine different materials to add sophistication and interest. For instance, pair a basic cotton tee with a leather jacket or a silk scarf. This contrast in textures can make an outfit more dynamic without relying on color or pattern.

Play with Proportions:

Balance fitted basics with oversized statement items. A fitted turtleneck can be paired with wide-leg patterned pants for a modern silhouette. This play with proportions can create a visually appealing and balanced look.

Color Coordination:

Use color to create harmony in your outfit. Match a statement piece with a basic item in complementary shades to achieve a cohesive look. This technique helps in tying the outfit together and ensuring that the statement piece enhances rather than overwhelms.

Layering:

Layering basics with statement pieces adds complexity and dimension to your look. A simple dress can be enhanced with a bold jacket or an oversized scarf. Layering allows for creativity and adaptability, especially in transitional weather.

Practical Tips

Invest in Quality Basics:

High-quality basics provide a reliable foundation and tend to last longer, ensuring they can support various statement pieces over time.

Edit Your Wardrobe Regularly:

Regularly assess your wardrobe to remove items that no longer fit your style, making room for new statement pieces that can refresh and revitalize your look.

Experiment and Explore:

Don't be afraid to try new combinations and push the boundaries of your style. Fashion is about exploration and finding what uniquely works for you, so take risks and have fun with your choices.

Balance Is Key:

Always aim for balance in your outfits. If your statement piece is particularly bold, keep your makeup and hairstyle more subdued to maintain harmony.

Consider the Occasion:

Tailor your use of statement pieces to the context. For a professional setting, opt for subtle statement accessories, while for social events, you can be more adventurous.

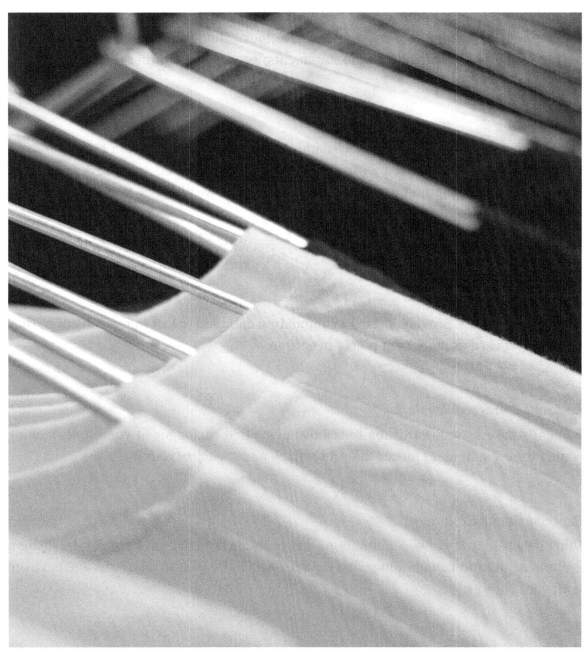

By thoughtfully combining basics with statement pieces, you can create a wardrobe that is both functional and expressive. This approach allows your unique style to shine through, offering endless possibilities for every occasion, and ensuring you always have something perfect to wear.

Building a Capsule Wardrobe

A capsule wardrobe is a thoughtfully curated collection of essential clothing items designed to maximize versatility and style while minimizing clutter. The concept focuses on quality over quantity, allowing for a streamlined and efficient approach to dressing. Here's a comprehensive guide to building your own capsule wardrobe:

Understanding the Concept

At its core, a capsule wardrobe comprises a limited number of timeless, high-quality pieces that can be mixed and matched to create a wide variety of outfits. This approach not only simplifies your wardrobe but also enhances your personal style.

Steps to Build a Capsule Wardrobe

Assess Your Lifestyle:

Evaluate your daily activities and wardrobe needs. Consider the environments you frequent—whether it's a corporate office, casual settings, or formal events. Your capsule wardrobe should align with your lifestyle to ensure practicality and functionality.

Define Your Style:

Reflect on your personal style preferences. Are you drawn to classic, minimalist, or eclectic styles? This understanding will guide your selections and ensure your wardrobe feels authentic to you.

Choose a Color Palette:

Select a cohesive color palette to ensure all pieces can be easily mixed and matched. Start with neutral tones like black, white, gray, navy, and beige, which serve as versatile bases. Incorporate a few accent colors that complement your skin tone and personal style for added interest.

Select Key Pieces:

Focus on building a foundation with essential items such as:

Tops: A classic white shirt, a neutral t-shirt, and a versatile blouse.

Bottoms: Quality denim jeans, tailored trousers, and a versatile skirt.

Outerwear: A well-fitted blazer, a timeless trench coat, and a seasonal jacket.

Dresses: A little black dress and a casual day dress.

Footwear: Comfortable flats, versatile heels, and a pair of sneakers.

Accessories: A reliable handbag, a statement necklace, and a scarf.

Incorporate Seasonal Items:

Add a few pieces to adapt to seasonal changes. For example, include a cozy sweater for winter or a lightweight cardigan for spring. This ensures your wardrobe remains practical year-round.

Limit the Number of Items:

Aim for around 30-40 pieces, including shoes and accessories. This encourages creativity in outfit combinations and keeps your wardrobe manageable. The exact number can vary based on personal preference, but the focus should remain on versatility and quality.

Focus on Quality Over Quantity:

Invest in high-quality pieces that are durable and timeless. Look for well-made garments with quality fabrics and craftsmanship. These items will withstand wear and tear, reducing the need for frequent replacements.

Regularly Edit Your Wardrobe:

Periodically review your capsule wardrobe. Remove items that no longer fit, suit your style, or serve your needs. Replace them with pieces that enhance your collection. This practice keeps your wardrobe relevant and aligned with your evolving style.

Add Personal Touches:

Incorporate a few statement pieces or accessories that reflect your personality. Whether it's a bold scarf, vintage jewelry, or a unique bag, these elements ensure your capsule wardrobe feels uniquely yours.

Benefits of a Capsule Wardrobe

Simplifies Decision Making:
With fewer pieces, selecting an outfit becomes quicker and less stressful, freeing up time for other priorities.

Saves Time and Money:
Investing in quality, timeless pieces reduce the need for frequent shopping, saving money in the long run.

Encourages Sustainability:
A smaller, more thoughtful wardrobe reduces waste and supports sustainable fashion practices, contributing to an eco-friendlier lifestyle.

Enhances Personal Style:
By focusing on pieces you love and that suit your lifestyle, you refine your personal style and feel more confident in your clothing choices.

By building a capsule wardrobe, you create a cohesive, stylish collection that serves you well in any situation. This approach not only simplifies your life but also elevates your style, allowing you to express yourself effortlessly with minimal effort. Embrace the freedom and creativity that comes with having a thoughtfully curated wardrobe tailored to your unique needs and preferences.

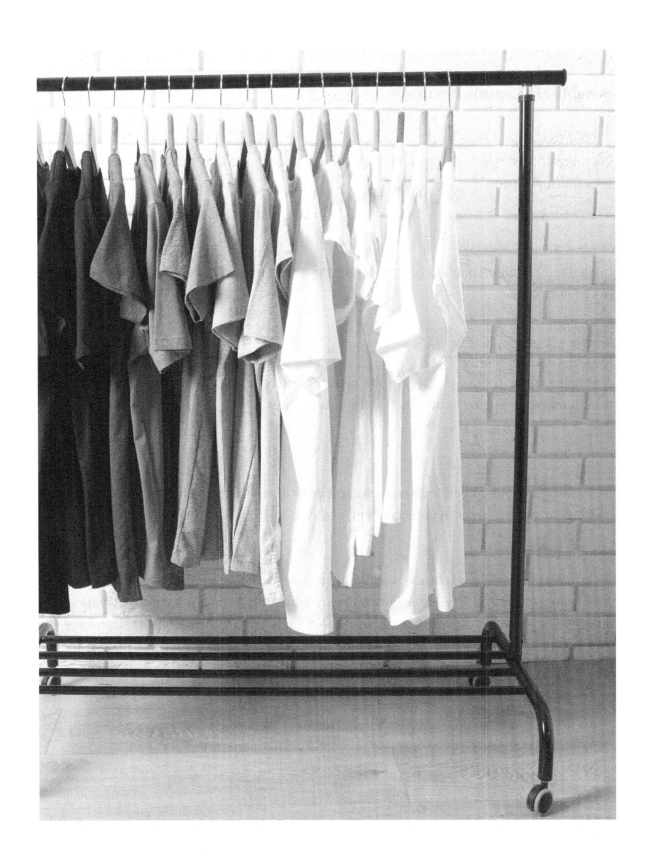

Adapting Your Wardrobe Seasonally

Adapting your wardrobe to the changing seasons ensures both comfort and style throughout the year. This process involves thoughtful adjustments to fabrics, colors, and layers, allowing your capsule wardrobe to remain versatile and functional.

Understanding Seasonal Needs

Each season brings unique weather conditions and style opportunities. Adapting your wardrobe means selecting appropriate materials, colors, and layering techniques to stay comfortable while maintaining your personal style.

Strategies for Seasonal Adaptation

Layering Basics:

Layering is key to adjusting for temperature fluctuations. In cooler months, layer a cozy sweater over a lightweight shirt or add a scarf for warmth. Consider layering a turtleneck under a dress for added warmth. In warmer months, opt for breathable fabrics and lighter layers, such as a camisole under a linen blouse.

Incorporate Seasonal Fabrics:

Choose fabrics that suit the season. Wool, cashmere, and fleece are ideal for winter, providing warmth and insulation. In summer, prioritize cotton, linen, and silk for their breathability and comfort. These materials ensure you remain comfortable and functional throughout seasonal changes.

Adjust Your Color Palette:

Transition your color palette to reflect the season's mood. In winter, opt for deeper, richer tones like burgundy, navy, and forest green to evoke warmth. Spring and summer call for brighter, lighter colors such as pastels like lavender and mint, or bold primary hues like coral and turquoise.

Swap Key Pieces:

Rotate specific items in and out of your wardrobe based on the season. For example, replace heavy coats with lighter jackets or cardigans in spring. Swap sandals and espadrilles for boots and closed-toe shoes as fall approaches. This rotation keeps your wardrobe fresh and seasonally appropriate.

Update Accessories:

Accessories are a simple way to adapt your wardrobe. In winter, add hats, gloves, and scarves for extra warmth, choosing materials like wool or cashmere. In summer, switch to sunglasses, sun hats, and lightweight scarves made from cotton or silk. These adjustments can dramatically alter the look and feel of your outfits.

Footwear Adjustments:

Change your footwear to suit the season. Boots are perfect for fall and winter, providing warmth, protection, and style. In contrast, sandals, loafers, and sneakers are ideal for spring and summer, offering comfort and breathability.

Consider Special Occasions:

Plan for seasonal events and holidays by incorporating appropriate attire. For winter holidays, consider a festive dress or a tailored suit with elegant accessories. Summer weddings or outdoor events might call for a lightweight dress or a linen suit.

Maintain Versatility:

Ensure that most pieces can transition between seasons with minor adjustments. A neutral trench coat, for example, can be layered for warmth in winter with a sweater and scarf or worn over a light dress in spring for a chic, polished look.

Organize Your Wardrobe:

Regularly reorganize your wardrobe to make seasonal items easily accessible. Store off-season clothing in bins or at the back of your closet and bring forward items suitable for the current season. This keeps your wardrobe organized and efficient.

Benefits of Seasonal Adaptation

Maximizes Wardrobe Efficiency:
Rotating items seasonally ensure that you make the most of your wardrobe without overcrowding it.

Enhances Comfort and Style:
Wearing seasonally appropriate clothing keeps you comfortable and ensures a polished appearance.

Encourages Creativity:
Adapting to each season allows for creativity in styling and experimenting with different looks, keeping fashion choices fresh and exciting.

By thoughtfully adapting your wardrobe seasonally, you maintain a stylish, functional, and cohesive collection all year round. This approach not only maximizes the potential of your capsule wardrobe but also keeps your fashion choices aligned with the changing seasons, ensuring both practicality and elegance.

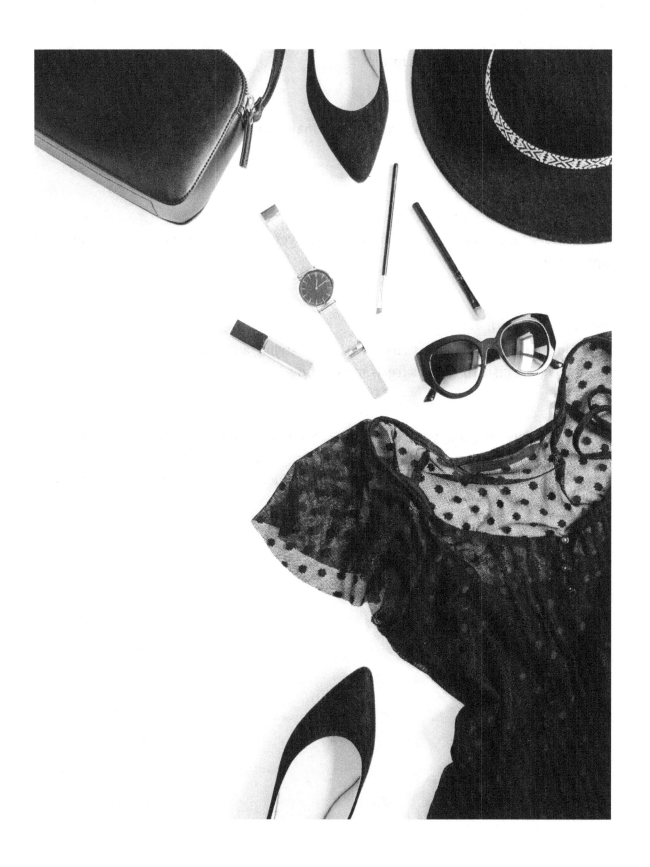

Chapter 4:

Understanding

Color and Patterns

Basics of Color Theory

Color is a fundamental element in design and art, influencing emotions, perceptions, and decisions. Mastering color theory empowers you to create compelling and harmonious compositions. This chapter delves into the essentials of color theory and the role of patterns.

The Color Wheel

The color wheel is a circular diagram representing the relationships between colors. It consists of:

Primary Colors:

Red, blue, and yellow. These cannot be created by mixing other colors and serve as the foundation.

Secondary Colors:

Green, orange, and purple, formed by mixing primary colors. For example, blue and yellow make green.

Tertiary Colors:

These are created by mixing a primary color with a neighboring secondary color, resulting in hues like red-orange and blue-green.

Color Harmony

Achieving color harmony is essential for creating visually appealing designs. Harmonious color combinations are pleasing to the eye and can be achieved through various schemes:

Complementary Colors:

Located opposite each other on the color wheel, such as red and green or blue and orange. These pairs offer high contrast and are ideal for making elements stand out.

Analogous Colors:

Found next to each other on the wheel, like yellow, yellow-green, and green. This scheme provides a serene and cohesive look, often found in nature.

Triadic Colors:

Three colors evenly spaced on the wheel, such as red, yellow, and blue. This scheme offers vibrant and balanced results, perfect for dynamic designs.

Monochromatic Colors:

Variations in lightness and saturation of a single hue. This approach creates a cohesive and soothing appearance.

By using the color wheel, you can craft harmonious outfits. Complementary colors, opposite each other on the wheel, create vibrant looks, while analogous colors, adjacent on the wheel, offer a more subtle harmony. These combinations can be used to emphasize or soften certain features.

Color Context and Perception

The perception of color can change based on its context. A color might appear different against various backgrounds or in different lighting conditions. Understanding this can help you manipulate how colors interact and ensure the desired visual impact.

Contrast:

High contrast between colors can make elements stand out, while low contrast can create a more subdued look. High-intensity colors are bright and striking, perfect for making bold fashion statements. Low-intensity colors are more muted and versatile, ideal for creating a subtle elegance.

Surrounding Colors:

Colors are affected by adjacent hues, which may alter their appearance. Consider the entire palette to maintain balance.

Color Value:

It describes the lightness or darkness of a color. Light colors can make you appear larger, while dark colors can have a slimming effect. Understanding how to balance intensity and value can help you create outfits that are visually interesting and flattering.

Warm vs. Cool Colors:

Warm and cool colors:

Warm colors (reds, oranges, yellows) evoke warmth and excitement, often associated with energy and positivity. Cool colors (blues, greens, purples), on the other hand, are calming and serene, often linked to tranquility and professionalism.

Skin tone:

Understanding your skin tone is crucial in choosing colors that enhance your natural beauty. Warm skin tones generally glow in warm colors, while cool skin tones are flattered by cool hues. Knowing your undertone can guide you in selecting clothes that make you look vibrant and healthy.

Psychological Effects of Color

Colors can evoke specific emotions and associations, influencing mood and behavior:

Red:

Often associated with passion, excitement, and urgency. It can stimulate energy but may also signify danger.

Blue:

Conveys calmness, trust, and stability. It is frequently used in corporate designs to evoke reliability.

Green:

Represents nature, growth, and harmony. It is soothing and can signify health and tranquility.

Yellow:

Evokes happiness, energy, and warmth. However, it can also caution or overwhelm if overused.

Understanding these psychological effects allows you to tailor designs to elicit desired emotional responses. Leveraging the psychological impact of colors can help you dress appropriately for different occasions. Choose colors that align with the impression you wish to make, whether it's confidence in a business meeting, for example, or warmth at a social gathering.

Patterns and Their Impact

Patterns play an integral role in fashion design, adding depth, texture, and character to garments. When selecting and combining patterns, consider the following:

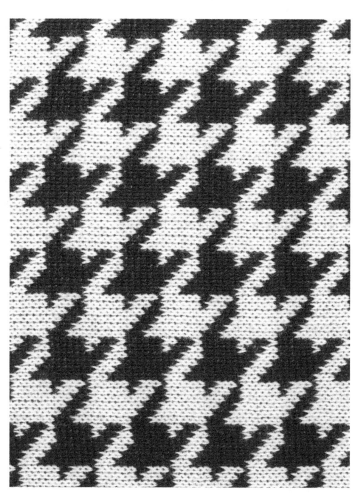

Consider Scale:

The scale of a pattern can significantly impact the overall look of a garment. Large patterns can be bold and eye-catching, making a statement, while smaller patterns tend to be more subtle and versatile.

Mixing Patterns:

Combining different patterns requires careful consideration of color and scale to avoid clashing. Successful pattern mixing often relies on balancing busy designs with more subdued elements.

Cultural Significance:

Many patterns have cultural meanings or historical significance, which can add depth and storytelling to a design. Incorporating such patterns thoughtfully can enrich a collection's narrative.

Texture and Fabric:

The texture and type of fabric can influence how a pattern appears. A pattern on a silky fabric may look different than the same pattern on a textured material.

As you can see, by understanding and applying the basics of color theory, you can curate a wardrobe that not only fits your body but also embodies your personal style. Mix unexpected colors, try new patterns, and embrace what makes you feel most like yourself. Your style is a canvas, and color is a powerful medium to paint your story. Embrace the power of color and patterns to craft a unique fashion narrative that is unmistakably yours.

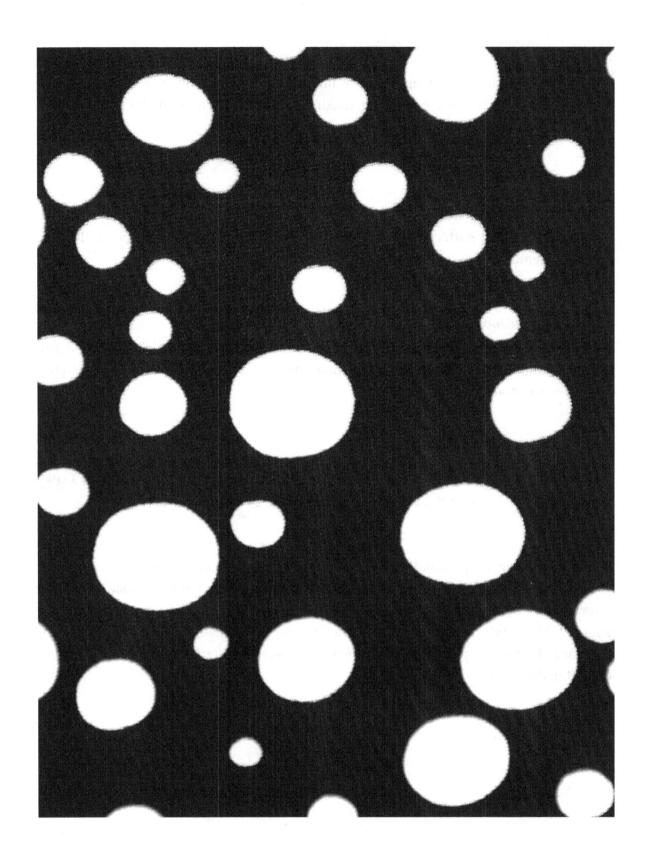

Discovering Your Personal Color Palette

Creating a personal color palette is a journey of self-expression and discovery. It involves selecting colors that resonate with you personally and align with your aesthetic goals.

Understanding Your Preferences

To start, examine your natural inclinations towards certain colors:

Emotional Response:

Consider how different colors affect your mood. Are you drawn to calming blues or invigorating reds? Reflect on which colors evoke positive emotions or memories.

Personal Associations:

Identify colors tied to meaningful experiences or cultural significance. Colors can carry personal or familial symbolism that adds depth to your choices.

Lifestyle and Environment:

Think about the environments you thrive in. Do you prefer the muted tones of a minimalist setting or the vibrant hues of a bustling cityscape?

Exploring Inspiration Sources

Gathering inspiration is key to expanding your palette possibilities:

Nature:

Nature is an abundant source of harmonious color combinations. Observe the subtle transitions of hues in a sunrise, the contrasting colors of a forest, or the vibrant palette of a coral reef.

Art and Design:

Explore museums, galleries, and online platforms. Analyze how artists and designers use color to convey emotion and narrative.

Fashion and Interiors:

Keep an eye on current trends, but also delve into historical color palettes from different eras and cultures for unique inspiration.

Experimenting with Combinations

Experimentation is crucial to discovering a unique palette:

Color Wheel Exploration:

Use the color wheel to explore complementary, analogous, and triadic schemes. This tool can help you understand how colors relate and contrast with one another.

Mood Boards:

Create physical or digital mood boards to test how your chosen colors interact. Include textures, fabrics, and images to see the overall effect.

Trial and Error:

Don't hesitate to adjust your selections. Testing shades in different lighting conditions can significantly affect their perception.

Making colors work for you

After exploring your personal color palette, we can now use another layer of color theory that serves as a guide for selecting clothing that enhances your natural features and aligns with your personal preferences, ultimately making fashion a means of elevating your looks while authentically expressing yourself.

Assess Your Skin Tone:

Start by identifying your skin tone—warm, cool, or neutral. This involves observing the undertones of your skin. Warm undertones typically have hints of yellow or gold, while cool undertones feature blue or pink hues. Neutral tones are a balance of both.

To determine your undertone, look at the veins on your wrist: if they appear greenish, you likely have warm undertones; if they appear bluish, you probably have cool undertones.

Consider Your Eye and Hair Color:

Your eye and hair color are key elements in selecting the right colors. Certain shades can enhance your eye color or create a striking contrast with your hair.

Experiment with colors to see which ones make your eyes sparkle or complement your hair. For instance, deep blues might highlight blue eyes, while rich auburn shades could enhance brown or red hair.

Lifestyle and Personal Preferences:

Your lifestyle and personal taste should inform your color palette. Think about the image you want to project and how colors can reflect your personality.

If you're outgoing and energetic, vibrant colors might resonate with you. For a more understated or professional appearance, classic neutrals may be preferable.

Building a Versatile Palette:

Create a balance of neutrals, statement colors, and accent hues. Neutrals like black, white, grey, and beige are versatile and form a solid foundation. Statement colors, such as bold reds or deep blues, express your individuality. Accent hues can be used in accessories or smaller pieces for added interest.

This approach ensures your wardrobe is cohesive and versatile, allowing for easy mixing and matching across different outfits and occasions.

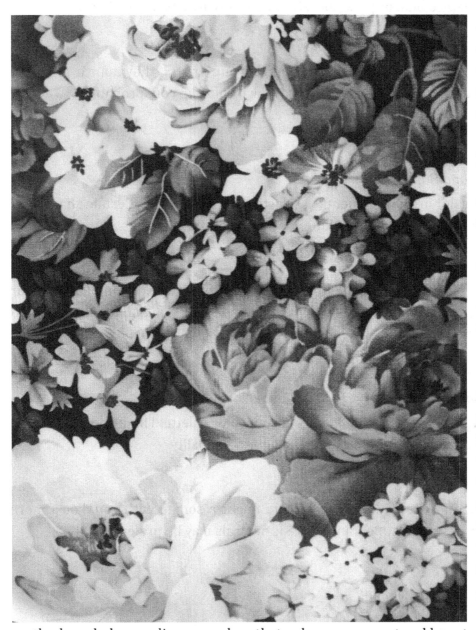

Seasonal Color Analysis:
Consider using seasonal color analysis, which categorizes palettes into seasons—spring, summer, autumn, and winter—based on the color characteristics that suit you best.

Spring and autumn palettes typically feature warm, earthy tones, while summer and winter palettes include cooler, more vibrant colors. This structured method can help you discover colors that enhance your natural beauty all year round.

Psychological Impact of Colors:
Different colors evoke different emotions and can influence how you feel and how others perceive you. Understanding this psychological impact can guide your choices.

For example, wearing blue might evoke calmness and reliability, while yellow can convey optimism and energy. Use this knowledge to select colors that align with your mood and desired impression.

Experiment and Adapt:

Discovering your personal color palette is an ongoing journey. Don't be afraid to experiment with new colors and patterns as your tastes and circumstances evolve.

Personal style is dynamic, and your palette should adapt to reflect who you are at each stage of your life. As you grow, allow your color choices to evolve with you.

Practical Application:

Once you've identified your palette, apply it practically by organizing your wardrobe around these colors. This can simplify shopping and outfit planning, ensuring everything in your closet works well together.

Invest in key pieces in your best colors and use seasonal trends to refresh your wardrobe without deviating from your core palette.

By discovering and embracing your personal color palette, you can curate a wardrobe that not only complements your physical features but also resonates with your personality and lifestyle. This thoughtful approach to color helps you express yourself authentically and confidently through fashion, making every outfit a true reflection of who you are.

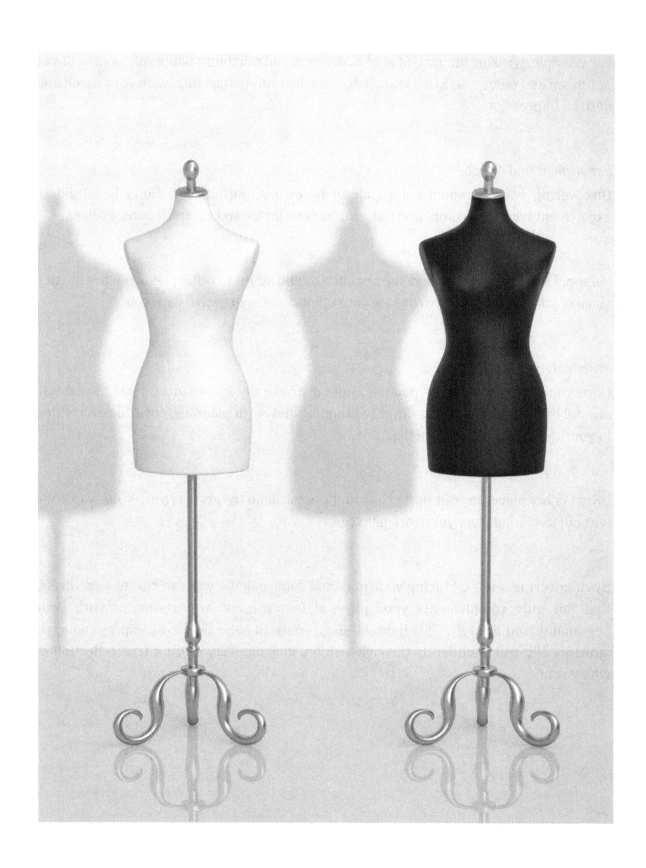

Incorporating Patterns and Textures into Outfits

Integrating patterns and textures into your wardrobe can significantly enhance your style, adding depth, interest, and personality to your outfits. Understanding how to mix and match these elements is key to creating a polished and cohesive look.

Understanding Patterns

Patterns are diverse and can range from subtle to bold, each bringing its own flair:

Stripes and Checks:

These timeless patterns offer versatility. Stripes can vary in direction and width, with vertical stripes elongating the silhouette and horizontal ones adding width. Checks, like plaids and gingham, provide a structured and classic look. Experiment with pairing different scales of stripes or checks for a modern twist.

Florals and Paisleys:

Often associated with a romantic or bohemian style, these patterns can range from delicate and intricate to bold and vibrant, allowing for seasonal adaptability. Florals can be tropical, vintage, or abstract, each offering a distinct mood.

Geometric and Abstract:

These patterns offer a modern edge, perfect for making a statement or adding a contemporary touch. They can be symmetrical or freeform, adding variety to your wardrobe. Consider using geometric patterns in minimalist or monochromatic outfits for a chic look.

Animal Prints:

From leopard to zebra, these prints add a wild, adventurous element to any outfit. They can act as a neutral, pairing well with many colors. Use animal prints sparingly for a sophisticated touch or boldly for a statement piece.

Mixing Patterns

Combining patterns can be bold but rewarding when balanced correctly:

Scale and Proportion:

Mixing patterns of different scales can prevent a cluttered look. For instance, pairing a large floral with a small stripe creates visual harmony. Think about the visual weight each pattern carries and adjust accordingly.

Color Coordination:

Ensure that the patterns share a common color palette or complementary hues to maintain cohesion. This makes even bold combinations appear intentional and stylish. A cohesive color scheme can unify disparate patterns.

Neutral Base:

Use neutral pieces to anchor patterned items, allowing them to stand out as focal points without overwhelming the outfit. Neutrals can soften bold patterns, making them more wearable.

Pattern Hierarchy:

Choose one dominant pattern and support it with a secondary, subtler pattern to maintain balance. This approach helps guide the eye and creates a focal point.

Understanding Textures

Textures add a tactile dimension to outfits, enhancing their visual and sensory appeal:

Knit and Wool:

These cozy textures are perfect for adding warmth and comfort, ideal for layering in cooler months or creating a relaxed, casual look. Experiment with chunky knits or fine merino wool for different effects.

Silk and Satin:

Smooth and lustrous, these textures add elegance and sophistication. They are perfect for formal occasions or adding a luxurious touch to a casual outfit. Consider silk for blouses and satin for evening wear.

Leather and Denim:

These sturdy textures provide a rugged, durable look, adding edge and versatility. Leather can be sleek and polished, while denim offers a classic, casual vibe. Use these textures in jackets, pants, or accessories for a timeless appeal.

Lace and Embroidery:

Delicate textures that add a feminine and intricate element to any ensemble, suitable for both casual and formal settings. Incorporate lace in tops or dresses and embroidery in outerwear for added detail.

Combining Textures

Layering different textures can create a rich and dynamic outfit:

Contrasting Textures:

Pairing rough textures like tweed with smooth ones like silk creates a balanced contrast, adding interest without clashing. This approach highlights each texture's unique qualities.

Layering:

Use varied textures in layers, such as a chunky knit over a silk blouse, to add depth and complexity without bulk. Layering also allows for practical adaptation to changing weather.

Monochrome Variations:

Using different textures within the same color palette can create a sophisticated and cohesive look. This technique adds interest while maintaining elegance.

Accessories as Accents

Accessories offer an excellent way to introduce patterns and textures subtly:

Scarves and Ties:

These can introduce patterns like paisleys or polka dots, adding a pop of interest without overwhelming the outfit. They are versatile and can be easily swapped to refresh an outfit.

Bags and Shoes:

Incorporate textures like leather, suede, or metallic finishes to add dimension. A patterned bag or textured shoe can act as a statement piece and elevate a simple outfit.

Jewelry:

Use statement pieces with textured finishes or intricate patterns to enhance your outfit. Bold jewelry can add sparkle and interest, drawing attention to specific areas.

Personal Style and Confidence

Ultimately, incorporating patterns and textures is about expressing your personal style:

Confidence:

Wear what makes you feel strong and authentic. Your comfort with patterns and textures will reflect in your confidence. Confidence can transform an outfit from good to great.

Experimentation:

Don't be afraid to try new combinations. Fashion is exploration, and discovering what works best for you is part of the exciting journey. Embrace trial and error as a learning experience.

Signature Style:

Develop a signature look by consistently incorporating certain patterns or textures that resonate with you. This can help create a personal brand and make dressing easier and more enjoyable.

Adaptability:

Be open to evolving your style as trends change and your tastes develop. Patterns and textures offer endless possibilities to refresh your wardrobe without a complete overhaul.

By thoughtfully incorporating patterns and textures into your outfits, you can craft visually captivating looks that reflect your unique personality. Whether for everyday wear or special occasions, these elements can transform your wardrobe and elevate your fashion game, making every ensemble an opportunity for creative expression.

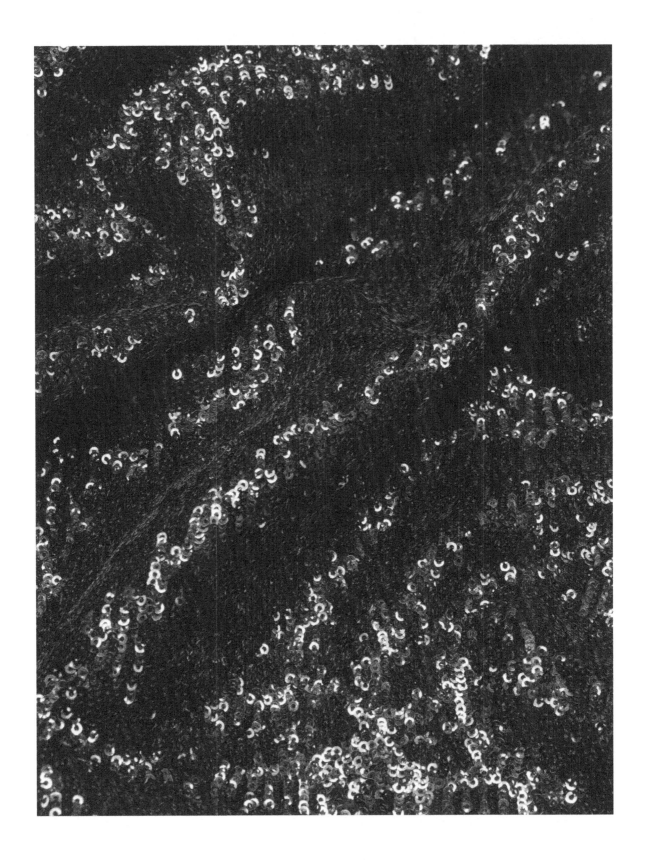

Balancing Bold and Neutral Tones

Achieving a harmonious balance between bold and neutral tones can elevate your outfits, allowing you to express creativity while maintaining sophistication. Understanding how to combine these elements effectively is key to versatile styling.

Understanding Bold Tones

Bold tones are vibrant and eye-catching, often used to make a statement:

Primary Colors:
Red, blue, and yellow add energy and interest. These foundational colors can be used as focal points, such as a red coat or a blue dress, and pair well with a variety of neutrals.

Jewel Tones:
Rich colors like emerald, sapphire, and ruby bring luxury and depth. They are perfect for adding sophistication to an outfit and can transition seamlessly from day to night.

Pastels and Neons:
While pastels offer a soft, muted appearance, neons are bright and flashy. Pastels can be used for a subtle pop of color, while neons are ideal for making a bold statement.

Earthy Bold Tones:
Colors like terracotta, mustard, and forest green add a warm, grounded feel, ideal for creating a cozy and inviting look.

The Role of Neutral Tones

Neutrals provide balance and grounding to bold tones:

Classic Neutrals:

Black, white, gray, and beige serve as a versatile base, allowing bold colors to stand out without overwhelming the outfit. They are timeless and can be paired with almost any color.

Earthy Neutrals:

Tones like olive, tan, and taupe add warmth and create a relaxed, natural look. They work well with both bold and muted hues, offering versatility.

Metallic Neutrals:

Silver, gold, and bronze can act as neutrals while adding a touch of elegance and shine to an outfit.

Combining Bold and Neutral Tones

Creating balance involves thoughtful pairing:

Focal Points:

Use bold tones to draw attention to specific areas, such as a statement jacket or vibrant shoes, while keeping the rest of the outfit neutral. This approach ensures a balanced look without overwhelming.

Layering:

Layer bold pieces over neutral basics to add interest without overpowering. For example, a bright scarf or colorful bag can enhance a neutral ensemble, adding depth and dimension.

Proportion:

Balance the proportion of bold and neutral elements. Too much bold can overwhelm, while too little may not have the desired impact. Aim for a harmonious blend that reflects your style.

Texture and Pattern:

Incorporate textured neutrals, like a knit sweater, with bold patterns to create a dynamic yet balanced outfit.

Transitioning Between Seasons

Use bold and neutral tones to adapt your wardrobe for different seasons:

Spring/Summer:

Incorporate lighter neutrals with pastel or bright bolds to reflect the freshness of the season. Think white pants with a bold floral top or a pastel blazer over a neutral dress.

Fall/Winter:

Opt for darker neutrals paired with jewel tones for a cozy, rich look. A charcoal coat with an emerald scarf creates a sophisticated ensemble that is both warm and stylish.

Year-Round Essentials:

Invest in pieces like a classic beige trench or a black blazer that can be paired with bold tones throughout the year.

Accessorizing with Bold and Neutral Tones

Accessories can subtly introduce or highlight bold tones:

Jewelry:

Use bold-colored jewelry to add a touch of vibrancy to a neutral outfit. Statement necklaces or earrings can transform a simple look into something extraordinary.

Footwear and Bags:

A brightly colored shoe or bag can act as a statement piece in an otherwise neutral ensemble. These accessories are versatile and can be easily swapped for different looks.

Belts and Hats:

These smaller accessories can introduce bold tones without overwhelming the entire look. A bold belt can accentuate your waist, while a colorful hat can add personality.

Personal Style and Confidence

Balancing bold and neutral tones is ultimately about personal expression:

Confidence:

Choose colors that make you feel empowered and comfortable. Confidence can make even the boldest outfits work seamlessly. Trust your instincts and wear what feels right.

Experimentation:

Don't hesitate to mix and match different combinations to discover what feels right for you. Fashion is about exploration and finding joy in self-expression. Try new pairings and step outside your comfort zone.

Developing a Signature Style:

Over time, find a balance that reflects your unique style. Whether you prefer more neutral looks with bold accents or vibrant outfits grounded by neutrals, embrace what makes you feel most like yourself.

By balancing bold and neutral tones, you can create versatile and stylish outfits that reflect your personality. This approach allows you to seamlessly transition between occasions and seasons, ensuring your wardrobe remains dynamic and engaging.

Chapter 5:

Dressing for Your

Body Type

Identifying Different Body Shapes

Understanding your body shape is essential for selecting clothing that enhances your natural silhouette. Each body type has unique characteristics, and knowing these can help you choose outfits that flatter your figure, boost your confidence, and express your personal style. Below, we'll explore the most common body shapes, how to identify them, and specific styling tips to make the most of your unique proportions.

Apple Shape

The apple shape is characterized by a fuller upper body, with broader shoulders and a larger bust. The waist is less defined, and weight is often carried around the midsection. To dress an apple-shaped body, it's important to create balance and elongate the torso.

Styling Tips:
Tops: Opt for A-line cuts, draped fabrics, or peplum tops that provide structure without clinging to the waist. V-necks or scoop necklines can elongate the neck and draw attention upward.

Dresses: Choose empire waistlines that highlight the bust while skimming over the midsection and consider wrap dresses that define the waist.

Bottoms: Straight-leg or boot-cut jeans can create a streamlined look. Avoid overly tight pants that may emphasize the midsection.

Pear Shape

A pear-shaped body features a narrower upper body with smaller shoulders and bust, and wider hips and thighs. The waist is typically well-defined, making it a key area to highlight.

Styling Tips:

Tops: Choose blouses with wide necklines, embellished details, or off-the-shoulder styles to draw attention to your upper body. Light colors and patterns can also help balance proportions.

Bottoms: A-line skirts and wide-leg pants are excellent choices as they skim over the hips. Darker colors on the bottom can create a more balanced look.

Dresses: Fit-and-flare dresses are perfect for accentuating the waist while providing a flattering silhouette for your hips.

Hourglass Shape

An hourglass figure has a well-defined waist, with nearly equal bust and hip measurements. This shape is often considered the ideal silhouette in fashion, and the key is to enhance your curves.

Styling Tips:

Tops: Fitted tops, wrap shirts, and tailored blazers can highlight the waist while celebrating your curves. Avoid boxy styles that can hide your shape.

Dresses: Opt for bodycon dresses or fitted styles that cinch at the waist. Belted dresses can also enhance the hourglass form.

Bottoms: High-waisted skirts and tailored trousers can accentuate your curves while providing a polished look.

Rectangle Shape

A rectangle shape is characterized by a straight silhouette with little definition at the waist. Shoulders, bust, and hips are typically similar in width, making it essential to create the illusion of curves.

Tops: Look for tops with ruffles, layers, or peplum details that add volume and dimension. Experiment with prints and textures to create visual interest.

Dresses: A-line dresses and fit-and-flare styles can help create a curvier silhouette. Avoid overly straight cuts that may not define the waist.

Bottoms: Utilize belted styles and wide-leg pants to create shape. High-waisted styles can also help define the waistline.

Inverted Triangle Shape

The inverted triangle shape features broad shoulders and a larger bust, with narrower hips and a less-defined waist. The key for this body type is to create balance by emphasizing the lower body.

Styling Tips:

Tops: Choose softer, flowing fabrics and avoid structured shoulder pads or overly embellished tops that can add bulk to the upper body. V-necks can help elongate the neckline.

Bottoms: Flared skirts, wide-leg pants, and palazzo trousers can create volume below the waist, balancing your proportions. A-line skirts are also flattering.

Dresses: Look for styles that draw attention to the legs, such as fit-and-flare dresses or those with interesting hemlines.

Identifying your body shape is the first step to dressing in a way that makes you feel confident and stylish. By understanding the characteristics of your body type, you can make informed choices that enhance your natural beauty. Remember, the most important factor in fashion is to wear what makes you feel good—embrace your shape and express your unique style!

Beyond identifying your body shape, consider your personal style preferences, lifestyle, and the occasions you dress for. Fashion is not just about fitting into a mold but about celebrating individuality. Accessories, color choices, and layering can all play a significant role in your overall look.

Experiment with different styles and don't be afraid to step out of your comfort zone. The right outfit can empower you and allow you to express who you are. Ultimately the journey of discovering your personal style is just as important as the destination.

Understanding Fabric and Fit

When dressing for your body type, the choice of fabric and fit is just as crucial as the cut and style of the clothing. Different fabrics drape differently on the body, influencing how an outfit looks and feels.

Fabrics:
Lightweight, flowing materials like chiffon or silk can create beautiful movement, while heavier fabrics like denim or canvas provide structure. Understanding what fabrics work best for your body type can enhance your overall appearance. For example, if you have an apple shape, opting for softer fabrics that drape can help create a flattering silhouette without adding bulk.

Fit:
Proper fit is essential for any body type. Ill-fitting clothes can detract from your appearance and comfort. Invest in tailoring when necessary to ensure your clothes fit perfectly. A well-tailored piece can transform your look and provide a polished finish.

Embracing Color and Patterns

Color and patterns are powerful tools in fashion. They can influence how your body shape is perceived and can help you express your personality.

Color Choices:

Dark colors tend to be slimming, while bright colors can attract attention. Use this to your advantage by wearing darker shades on areas you wish to downplay and brighter hues on areas you want to highlight. For example, pear shapes might wear darker colors on the bottom while opting for colorful or patterned tops.

Patterns:

Vertical stripes can elongate, while horizontal stripes can add width. Florals, polka dots, and geometric prints can also play a significant role in drawing attention to specific areas. Understanding how to use patterns can enhance your outfits and create a unique look that showcases your style.

Accessorizing for Your Shape

Accessories can elevate your outfit and help balance proportions. The right accessories can draw attention to your best features and add a personal touch to your ensemble.

Belts:

Using belts can highlight your waist, creating definition. A wide belt can be particularly flattering for hourglass and rectangle shapes, while a thinner belt can work well for pear shapes.

Jewelry:

Statement necklaces can draw the eye upward for apple shapes, while dangling earrings can enhance the features of inverted triangle shapes. Choose accessories that complement your body shape and enhance your overall look.

Footwear:

The right shoes can also impact how your outfit looks. For example, heels can elongate the legs, making them a great choice for all body types. Ankle boots or flats might be better suited for certain silhouettes, depending on how they balance your proportions.

Confidence is Key

Ultimately, the most vital aspect of dressing for your body type is confidence. No matter your shape, wearing clothes that make you feel good will shine through in your demeanor. Embrace your unique features and celebrate what makes you, you. The most stylish person in the room is often the one who exudes self-assurance.

In conclusion, understanding your body shape is a valuable tool in your fashion arsenal.

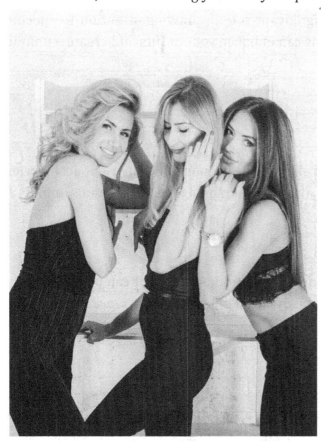

By identifying your shape and learning how to dress accordingly, you can create a wardrobe that enhances your natural beauty and reflects your personal style. Remember to consider fabric, fit, color, patterns, and accessories as you curate your outfits.

Fashion is not a one-size-fits-all approach; it's about finding what works best for you and having fun in the process. Embrace your individuality, experiment with different looks, and most importantly, wear what makes you feel empowered and beautiful. As you navigate the world of fashion, remember that the best accessory is always confidence—wear it with pride!

Tips for Flattering Fits

Finding the right fit is crucial for dressing well and feeling confident in your clothes. Here are some essential tips to help you achieve flattering fits for your body type:

Know Your Measurements

Before you shop, take the time to measure yourself accurately. Knowing your bust, waist, and hip measurements will help you choose clothing that fits properly. Keep these measurements handy when browsing online or in stores, as sizes can vary between brands.

Embrace Tailoring

Never underestimate the power of tailoring. If you find a piece you love but it doesn't fit perfectly, consider having it altered. A few simple adjustments can transform an ordinary item into something that fits like a glove. A well-tailored outfit not only looks polished but also enhances your natural shape.

Understand Proportions

Understanding how different clothing proportions affect your body shape is essential. For example, if you have a pear shape, wearing a fitted top with a flared skirt can create balance. Conversely, if you are an apple shape, pairing a looser top with structured bottoms can help define your silhouette. Experiment with different proportions to find what flatters you best.

Choose the Right Lengths

The length of your clothing can significantly impact your overall look. For instance, dresses and skirts that hit just above the knee can be universally flattering. Longer hemlines can elongate the body, while cropped styles can emphasize the waist. Consider your leg length and body proportions when choosing hemlines to create the most flattering effect.

Select the Right Silhouette

Each body shape benefits from specific silhouettes that enhance features. For instance:

A-Line:
This silhouette is great for pear shapes, as it skims over the hips while accentuating the waist.

Fit-and-Flare:
Perfect for hourglass figures, it hugs the waist and flares out over the hips.

Straight Cut:
Ideal for rectangle shapes, this silhouette provides a clean line and can create the illusion of curves.

Empire Waist:
Flattering for apple shapes, it draws attention to the bust while providing a flowing fit over the midsection.

Pay Attention to Straps and Sleeves

The style of straps and sleeves can greatly affect how clothing fits and flatters your body. For example:

Wide Straps:
These can help balance broader shoulders, making them a good choice for inverted triangle shapes.

Cap Sleeves:
These can add volume to the shoulders, which can be beneficial for pear shapes.

Three-Quarter Sleeves:
Great for all body types, they elongate the arms and create a sophisticated look.

Fabric Matters

The fabric you choose can impact how a garment fits and how it drapes on your body. Look for fabrics with some stretch, such as spandex or elastane blends, which can provide comfort and adaptability. Heavier fabrics like wool or denim can offer structure, while lighter fabrics like cotton or chiffon can create fluidity in your looks.

Experiment with Layers

Layering can enhance your outfit's fit and add dimension. For example, a fitted blazer over a loose top can create a balanced silhouette for apple shapes. Layering with cardigans or vests can also help define the waist for rectangle shapes. Just ensure that layers are not too bulky, as this can add unwanted volume.

Prioritize Comfort

While it's important to look good, comfort should never be compromised. Clothes that fit well should allow you to move freely and comfortably. If something feels restrictive or uncomfortable, it's likely not the right fit for you. Prioritize pieces that make you feel at ease; confidence shines brightest when you're comfortable in your skin.

Trust Your Instincts

Finally, trust your instincts when it comes to fit. If you feel fabulous in an outfit, wear it with pride, regardless of conventional fashion rules. Your personal style is about expressing who you are, and confidence is the best accessory you can wear.

Achieving a flattering fit is about more than just choosing the right size; it's about understanding your body and how different styles, fabrics, and fits can enhance your natural beauty. By knowing your measurements, embracing tailoring, and experimenting with proportions and silhouettes, you can curate a wardrobe that highlights your best features.

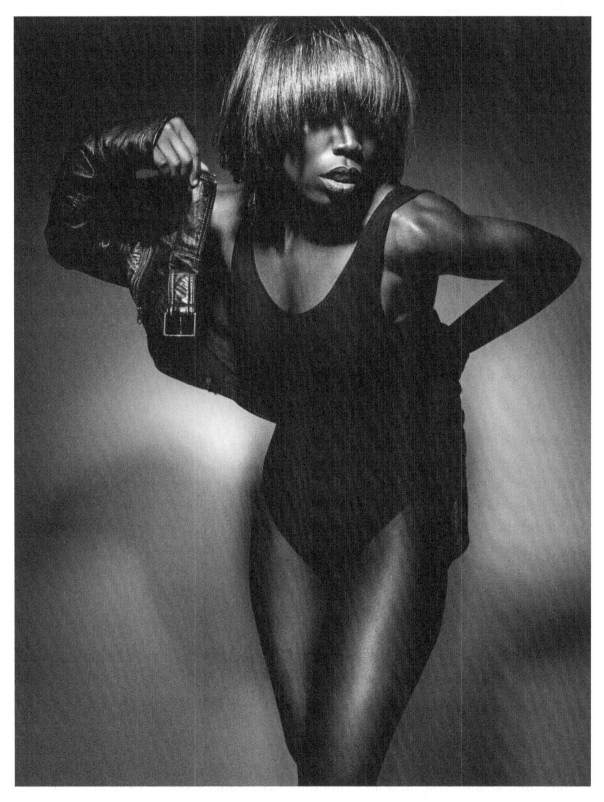

Emphasizing Your Best Features

When it comes to dressing for your body type, the ultimate goal is to highlight the features you love while creating a harmonious and balanced silhouette. Emphasizing your best attributes not only enhances your appearance but also boosts your confidence. Here are some comprehensive strategies to help you accentuate your best features:

Identify Your Best Features

Before you can emphasize your best features, you need to know what they are. Take a moment to stand in front of the mirror and assess your body. Is it your toned arms, defined waist, shapely legs, or lovely neckline that you adore? Understanding what you like about your body allows you to choose styles that showcase those areas. Consider what compliments you often receive or what makes you feel the most confident.

Use Color and Patterns Effectively

Colors and patterns are powerful tools in your wardrobe. Bright colors naturally draw the eye, so if you have stunning shoulders or a beautiful neckline, consider wearing off-the-shoulder tops or halter necklines in vibrant shades. Floral prints or bold patterns can also help highlight certain features. On the flip side, using darker colors or subtle patterns can be effective for areas you wish to downplay, creating a sense of balance in your overall look.

Tailoring is Key

Fit can make all the difference in how an outfit looks on you. Well-fitted clothing can transform your appearance and enhance your shape. Tailoring pieces to fit your unique dimensions can highlight your waistline, elongate your legs, or create a smooth line over your curves. For instance, a tailored blazer can cinch at the waist, creating an hourglass silhouette. Don't hesitate to invest in tailoring, as it can elevate even the simplest pieces in your wardrobe.

Layer Strategically

Layering is an excellent way to add depth and interest to your outfit while also emphasizing your best features. A fitted top under a flowy cardigan can highlight your figure while providing comfort. Use layers to create a structured look; for example, a structured jacket over a fitted dress can enhance your waistline. Be mindful of proportions—layering that is too bulky can overwhelm your frame, while strategically placed layers can create a flattering effect.

Accessorize Wisely

Accessories are not just embellishments; they can be key elements in emphasizing your best features. A statement necklace can draw attention to your neckline, making it a focal point. If you love your waist, a wide belt can cinch your waist while adding a pop of color or texture. Don't overlook the power of earrings and bracelets to frame your face and highlight your arms, respectively. Choose accessories that complement your outfit but also serve to accentuate your favorite features.

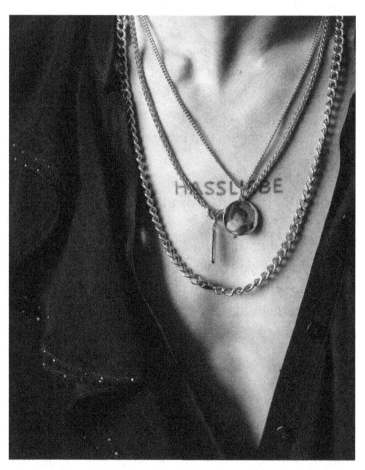

Choose Your Fabrics Carefully

The fabric of your clothing plays a significant role in how it drapes and fits your body. Lightweight, flowing materials can create a soft silhouette over curves, adding a sense of elegance. On the other hand, structured fabrics can provide support and shape where needed, such as in tailored trousers or blazers. Experiment with different textures—denim, chiffon, silk, and cotton can all behave differently on your body, so find what works best for the features you want to emphasize.

Footwear Matters

Don't underestimate the impact of footwear on your overall look. The right shoes can elongate your legs and complement your outfit beautifully. Heels can add height and create an elegant posture, enhancing your silhouette. If you prefer flats, choose styles that have a pointed toe to give the illusion of longer legs. Ankle boots can also be flattering when paired with the right hemline, providing a trendy yet sophisticated finish to your look.

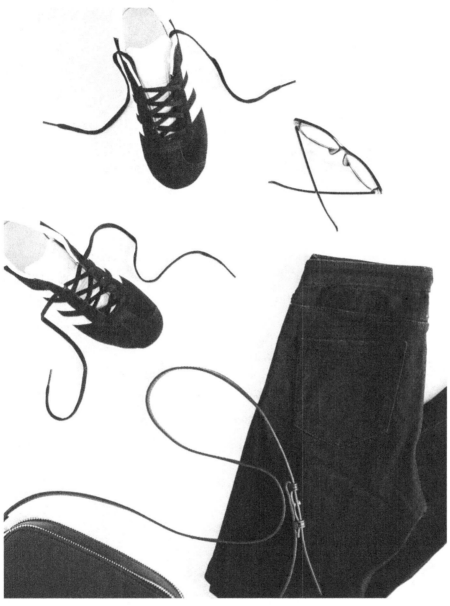

In conclusion, emphasizing your best features is about making thoughtful choices that celebrate your unique body shape. By understanding how to utilize color, fit, layering, and accessories, you can create outfits that not only look stunning but also make you feel empowered and confident.

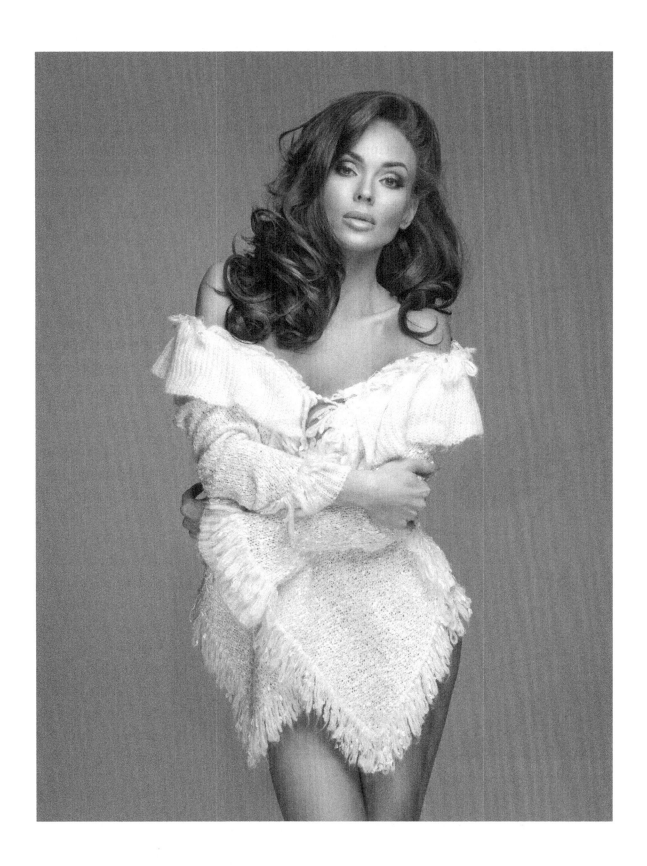

Dressing with Comfort and Confidence

Dressing well is not just about style; it's equally about comfort and confidence. When you feel comfortable in your clothing, it significantly boosts your self-esteem and allows you to present your best self to the world. Here are some essential strategies to help you dress in a way that maximizes both comfort and confidence:

Know Your Body's Needs

Understanding your body's unique needs is crucial for feeling comfortable. Consider factors like your body shape, size, and any specific features you may want to accommodate. For example, if you have a fuller bust, opt for tops with supportive structures like built-in bras or wider straps. If you have curvier hips, high-waisted pants can provide comfort and support while accentuating your waist.

Choose the Right Fabrics

Fabric choice plays a vital role in comfort. Natural fibers like cotton, linen, and bamboo are breathable and soft against the skin, making them ideal for everyday wear. Stretchy materials, such as spandex or elastane blends, can offer flexibility and ease of movement. Avoid stiff or scratchy fabrics that can irritate your skin or restrict your movements. Always consider the climate; lightweight fabrics are better for warmer weather, while heavier options can provide comfort in colder months.

Prioritize Fit Over Fashion Trends

Trends come and go, but the right fit is timeless. When you prioritize fit, you ensure that your clothes flatter your body type, which in turn boosts your confidence. It's better to invest in a few well-fitting, classic pieces than to fill your wardrobe with ill-fitting trendy items. Take the time to try on different sizes and styles to find the perfect fit for your shape. Remember, a good tailor can work wonders in altering garments to achieve the ideal fit.

Incorporate Versatile Pieces

Versatile pieces can be the backbone of a comfortable and stylish wardrobe. Invest in items that can be dressed up or down, such as a classic blazer, basic shirts, tailored trousers, or a little black dress. These pieces allow you to transition seamlessly from day to night while maintaining comfort. Look for garments that can be mixed and matched with other items in your wardrobe to create multiple outfits without compromising on comfort.

Mind Your Footwear

Comfortable shoes are essential for feeling confident and at ease. Choose footwear that supports your feet and complements your outfit. Sneakers or stylish flats can be great for casual outings, while block heels provide height without sacrificing comfort. If you're on your feet all day, consider cushioned insoles or shoes designed for all-day wear. Remember, the right footwear can enhance your posture and overall appearance.

Embrace Your Personal Style

Expressing your personal style is key to feeling confident in what you wear. Take the time to explore what styles resonate with you, whether it's bohemian, classic, sporty, or eclectic. Curate a wardrobe that reflects your personality and makes you feel authentic. When you wear clothing that aligns with your style, you naturally exude confidence.

Layer for Comfort

Layering is not only stylish but also functional. It allows you to adjust your outfit according to changing temperatures throughout the day. Lightweight cardigans, denim jackets, or oversized shirts can be easily added or removed to enhance comfort. Choose layers that have a good drape and fit well, so you don't feel bulky or constrained.

Practice Positive Self-Talk

Confidence begins from within. Practice positive self-talk and affirmations that remind you of your worth and beauty. When you feel good about yourself mentally, it is reflected in your outward appearance. Stand tall, maintain good posture, and embrace your unique features. As highlighted before, confidence is often the most attractive accessory you can wear.

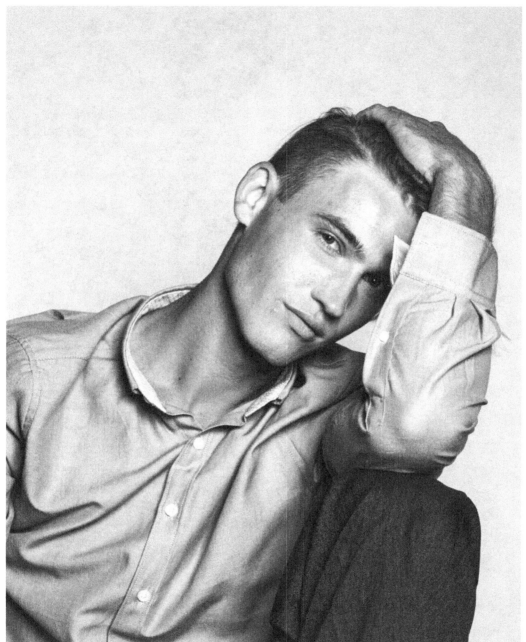

Dressing with comfort and confidence is about finding the right balance between style and ease. By understanding your body's needs, choosing the right fabrics, and prioritizing fit, you can create outfits that make you feel amazing. Embrace your personal style, invest in versatile pieces, and always remember that confidence shines through when you feel comfortable in your own skin. Celebrate your individuality, and let your confidence radiate through your clothing choices!

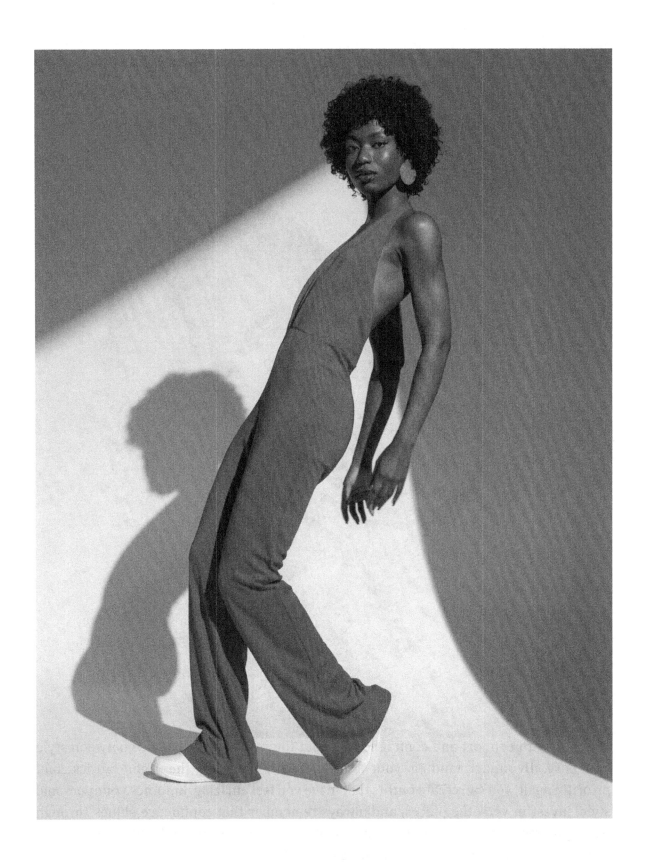

Chapter 6:

Accessorizing

Effectively

Key Accessories for Every Wardrobe

Accessorizing is the art of enhancing your outfit with thoughtful details that reflect your personal style. The right accessories can transform a simple look into something extraordinary, adding flair and individuality. In this chapter, we'll explore key accessories that every wardrobe should include, ensuring you're prepared for any occasion while also allowing your personality to shine through.

Statement Jewelry

A bold piece of jewelry can serve as the focal point of your outfit. Statement necklaces, oversized earrings, and chunky bracelets can instantly elevate even the most basic attire. These pieces act as conversation starters and can convey a lot about your personality. When selecting statement jewelry, consider your style—do you prefer bohemian, modern, or vintage vibes?

For a chic look, pair a statement necklace with a simple white tee and jeans, or wear oversized earrings with a sleek bun to draw attention to your face. Experiment with layering necklaces of varying lengths for a trendy, boho look or stack bracelets for a fun, eclectic vibe. Remember, the key is to balance bold pieces with understated clothing to avoid overwhelming your outfit.

Versatile Handbags

A well-chosen handbag can function as both a practical item and a style statement. Opt for a classic tote or a chic crossbody bag that works for various settings, from the office to dinner dates. When selecting a handbag, consider the size, shape, and color. Neutral colors like black, beige, or navy can seamlessly integrate into your wardrobe, making them easy to pair with countless outfits.

On the other hand, a bright or patterned bag can add a fun twist to your ensembles. Don't shy away from experimenting with seasonal trends as well; a vibrant handbag in a rich autumn hue can refresh your look during colder months. Consider also the functionality of your bags—look for options with pockets or compartments to keep your essentials organized.

Stylish Scarves

Scarves are incredibly versatile accessories that can be used in numerous ways. A lightweight scarf can be draped over your shoulders for a touch of elegance, while a thicker scarf can keep you warm in colder months. They can be tied around your neck, worn as a headband, or even used as a belt for a unique twist.

When choosing scarves, think about the fabric, color, and pattern. Silk scarves can add a luxurious touch, while knitted scarves are perfect for winter layering. Choose patterns and colors that can easily mix and match with your outfits, ensuring they remain a staple in your wardrobe. A vibrant print can add excitement to a monochrome outfit, while a classic plaid scarf can lend a timeless appeal.

Classic Footwear

Footwear can make or break an outfit. Investing in a few classic pairs that suit various occasions is essential—think sleek pumps for formal events, comfortable flats for everyday wear, and versatile ankle boots that can transition from day to night.

When selecting footwear, prioritize comfort without sacrificing style. Look for quality materials that offer support, especially if you'll be on your feet for long periods. Experimenting with different heel heights and styles can also add variety to your wardrobe. A pair of stylish sneakers can provide a casual yet trendy option, perfect for weekend outings or travel.

Timeless Sunglasses

A pair of stylish sunglasses can elevate any outfit while providing protection from the sun. Look for frames that flatter your face shape—cat-eye, aviators, or oversized designs can each make a bold statement. Sunglasses are not just a summer accessory; they can be a chic addition year-round.

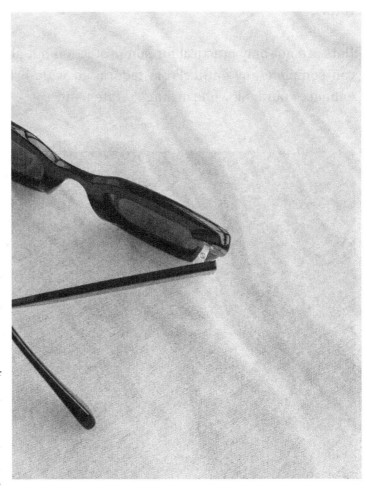

Choose lenses that offer UV protection to ensure your eyes are safeguarded from harmful rays. Sunglasses can add an air of mystery and sophistication to your look, making them a must-have for any fashion-forward individual. Pair them with a sundress for a relaxed summer vibe or with a leather jacket for a more edgy look.

Belts

Belts are often overlooked but can be a game changer in creating shape and definition in your outfits. A simple leather belt can clinch a loose dress or oversized top, instantly creating a flattering silhouette.

When selecting belts, consider different widths and materials. A thin belt can add a delicate touch to a flowy dress, while a wide belt can make a bold statement with a structured outfit. Don't be afraid to experiment with colors and textures—woven belts can add an earthy feel, while metallic belts can introduce a touch of glam.

Hats

Hats are not only practical for sun protection but also serve as a stylish accessory that can complete any outfit. From fedoras to wide-brimmed sun hats, the right hat can enhance your look while making a statement.

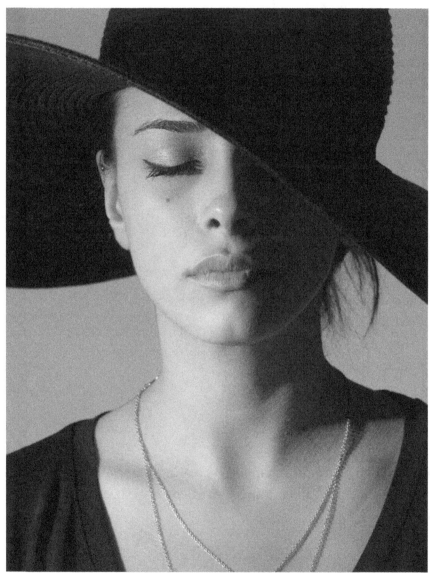

Consider the occasion when choosing a hat—beach outings call for floppy sun hats, while casual outings may suit a stylish baseball cap. Experimenting with different styles can reveal new facets of your fashion sense and provide an easy way to express yourself.

Layering Pieces

Layering pieces, such as cardigans, vests, and lightweight jackets, are essential accessories that can add depth to your outfits. These items not only provide warmth but also create visual interest. A well-fitted blazer can elevate a casual ensemble, while a long cardigan can add a relaxed touch to a more polished look.

When layering, consider the length and texture of each piece to ensure a harmonious balance. Mixing materials like denim, cotton, and knits can create a rich, dynamic outfit.

Don't shy away from layering different colors and patterns; just be mindful to keep the overall look cohesive.

Brooches and Pins

Brooches and pins are making a comeback as playful, vintage-inspired accessories. These small yet impactful pieces can be attached to jackets, bags, or even scarves, adding a personal touch to your look. Choose designs that resonate with your personality—floral motifs, quirky shapes, or elegant gems can all convey different aspects of your style.

Brooches are particularly effective for transforming classic pieces. Pinning one to a tailored blazer can add a touch of whimsy, while a cluster of pins on a simple bag can create a personalized statement.

Watches

A stylish watch is more than just a way to tell time; it's a statement accessory that can convey sophistication and elegance. Whether you prefer a classic leather band, a sleek metal bracelet, or a modern smartwatch, the timepiece you choose can reflect your lifestyle and taste.

Consider your daily activities when selecting a watch. A sporty design might be perfect for an active lifestyle, while a minimalist watch can complement a professional outfit. A well-chosen watch can effortlessly enhance your overall look, making it an essential accessory.

Accessorizing is not just about adding elements to your outfit; it's about expressing who you are and how you want to be perceived. The right accessories can elevate your look, making you feel more confident and stylish. Take the time to curate a collection of key accessories that resonate with your personal aesthetic, and don't hesitate to experiment and mix and match.

Remember, the beauty of accessorizing lies in its versatility. Each piece you choose holds the potential to transform your outfit, telling a story about your unique sense of style.

Embrace the art of accessorizing and let your creativity flow. With the right accessories, you can effortlessly turn any outfit into a reflection of your individuality, ensuring that you always step out in confidence and style.

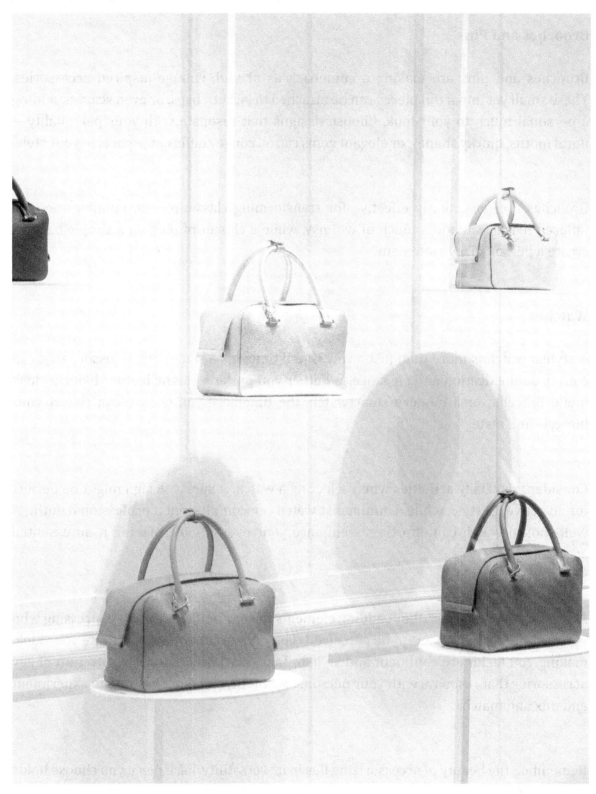

Statement Pieces vs. Everyday Wear

When it comes to accessorizing, understanding the distinction between statement pieces and everyday wear is crucial. Each category serves a unique purpose in your wardrobe, allowing you to express your style in different contexts and moods. Knowing how to balance these elements can elevate your fashion game significantly.

Statement Pieces

Statement pieces are bold, eye-catching accessories designed to draw attention. These items often feature striking designs, unusual shapes, or vibrant colors. The purpose of a statement piece is to make a memorable impact, transforming an otherwise simple outfit into something extraordinary. Some examples are:

Chunky Necklaces: A large, ornate necklace can serve as the centerpiece of your look. Pair it with a simple top to let it shine.

Bold Earrings: Oversized hoops or elaborate chandelier earrings can frame your face beautifully and add a dramatic flair.

Unique Handbags: A handbag with an unconventional shape or pattern can serve as a conversation starter and can instantly elevate your outfit.

Styling Tips:
Keep the Rest Simple: When wearing a statement piece, it's best to keep the rest of your outfit relatively understated. This allows the accessory to shine without overwhelming your look.

Mix and Match with Care: If you choose to wear multiple statement pieces, ensure they complement each other. A good rule of thumb is to stick to one or two bold items and keep the rest of your accessories subtle.

Occasion Matters: Statement pieces are best suited for special occasions or events where you want to make a lasting impression. They can add a touch of glamour to parties, weddings, or nights out.

Everyday Wear

Everyday wear accessories are more versatile and practical. These items are typically subtler, designed for daily use and comfort. They enhance your outfit without stealing the spotlight, making them perfect for casual outings, work, or running errands. Here are some examples:

Simple Stud Earrings: A pair of classic studs can add a touch of elegance without being overpowering.

Basic Scarves: A lightweight scarf in a neutral color can add warmth and texture to your everyday outfits.

Classic Handbags: A structured tote or crossbody bag in a versatile color can carry your essentials while complementing various looks.

Styling Tips:
Mix and Match Freely: Everyday wear items can be combined with a variety of outfits. Feel free to mix different textures and colors to create a cohesive, stylish look.

Invest in Quality: Since these pieces will be worn frequently, invest in high-quality items that will stand the test of time both in terms of style and durability.

Personalize Your Look: Everyday wear doesn't have to be boring. Choose accessories that reflect your personality, whether through unique patterns, colors, or small embellishments.

Finding the Balance

The key to effective accessorizing lies in finding the right balance between statement pieces and everyday wear. Here are a few strategies to help you achieve this:

Assess Your Lifestyle:

Consider your daily activities and the types of outfits you typically wear. If you find yourself in casual settings most of the time, prioritize everyday wear while incorporating statement pieces for special occasions.

Layering Techniques:

You can create interest by layering both types of accessories. For example, wear a simple outfit topped with a statement necklace and complement it with understated earrings. This layering can create a well-rounded look.

Consider Versatility:

Some items can serve dual purposes. A bold ring might work as a statement piece at a party but can also add flair to a work outfit when styled correctly. Look for accessories that can transition between different settings.

Understanding the roles of statement pieces and everyday wear in your wardrobe is essential for effective accessorizing. By strategically incorporating both types of accessories, you can create outfits that are both practical and stylish. Remember, fashion is about expressing who you are, and the right accessories can help you do just that. Embrace the versatility of your wardrobe, and let your accessories tell your unique story, whether you're making a bold statement or enjoying the simplicity of everyday wear.

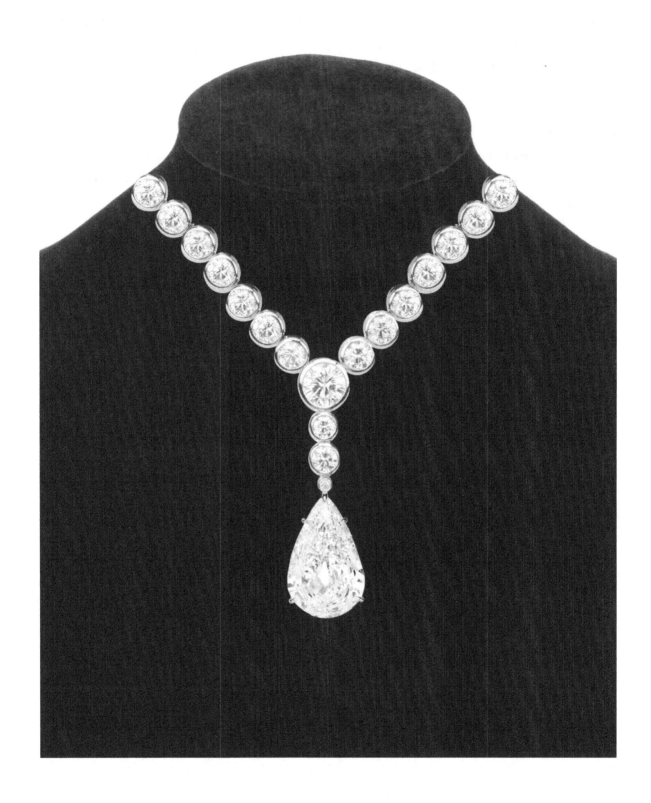

Incorporating Jewelry, Scarves, and Bags

As you can see, accessorizing is an art that can dramatically transform your look, adding personality and flair to even the simplest outfits. This section explores how to incorporate jewelry, scarves, and bags effectively, ensuring you create a harmonious and stylish ensemble.

Jewelry

Jewelry serves as a reflection of your personality and can enhance your outfit in numerous ways. Here are some tips to help you select and style your jewelry:

Statement vs. Delicate:

Statement Pieces: These bold items, such as oversized earrings or chunky necklaces, can serve as the focal point of your outfit. Pair them with simple clothing to let the jewelry shine. For instance, a vibrant statement necklace can elevate a plain white t-shirt and jeans.

Delicate Items: Subtle pieces, like thin rings or minimalist pendants, can add elegance without overpowering your look. They work wonderfully with layered outfits or intricate designs.

Layering Techniques:

Necklaces: Experiment with different lengths and styles. For a trendy layered look, mix a choker with longer chains, ensuring they vary in length to create visual interest.

Bracelets: Stack bangles, cuffs, and charm bracelets for a bohemian vibe. Consider mixing metals or textures for a more eclectic look but keep the overall color scheme in mind to maintain balance.

Occasion-Specific Choices:

For casual outings, opt for playful and colorful pieces that reflect your fun side. On the other hand, for professional settings, choose classic and understated jewelry, such as stud earrings or simple hoops, that convey sophistication and confidence.

In formal situations, consider timeless items like diamond studs or a pearl necklace, which exude elegance and class.

Personal Style:

Your jewelry should reflect your personal style. Whether you prefer vintage, bohemian, or modern pieces, select items that resonate with you. Don't hesitate to mix styles—wearing vintage earrings with a contemporary dress can create an interesting contrast.

Scarves

Scarves are incredibly versatile accessories that can enhance any outfit, providing warmth and style. Here are some tips on how to incorporate them effectively:

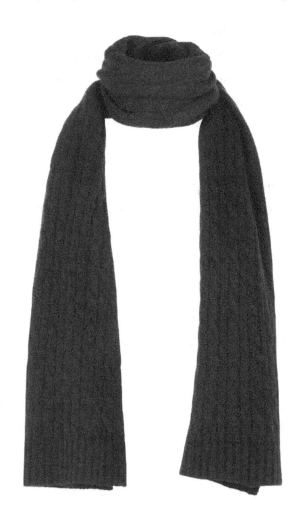

Tying Techniques:

The way you tie a scarf can change its entire look. Explore various methods, such as the classic loop, a chic knot, or a casual drape. You can even use scarves as belts or headbands, adding a creative spin to your outfit.

For a sophisticated look, try the Parisian knot, which involves folding the scarf in half, placing it around your neck, and pulling the ends through the loop.

Color and Pattern:

Scarves offer a fantastic opportunity to introduce color and pattern into your wardrobe. A floral scarf can add a cheerful touch to an otherwise muted outfit, while a striped or polka-dotted scarf can inject some fun.

When mixing patterns, ensure that at least one color ties them together. This creates a cohesive look despite the variety of designs.

Seasonal Choices:

In spring and summer, opt for lightweight fabrics like cotton or silk that drape beautifully and breathe easily. Bright colors and pastel shades can enhance your seasonal wardrobe.

In fall and winter, heavier materials such as wool or cashmere not only provide warmth but also add texture. A chunky knit scarf can become a cozy statement piece when paired with a simple coat.

Functionality:

Beyond aesthetics, consider the functionality of your scarf. A large scarf can double as a shawl during chilly evenings, while a lightweight scarf can serve as a wrap for sun protection.

Bags

Bags are essential accessories that combine practicality and style. Here's how to choose and use them effectively:

Size Matters:

When selecting a bag, consider the size in relation to your outfit. A small clutch is perfect for evening events, while a medium-sized crossbody bag is great for casual outings or running errands. Oversized totes are ideal for work or travel, offering ample space without compromising style.

Color Coordination:

Your bag can either match or contrast with your outfit. A neutral-colored bag can seamlessly blend with any look, while a bright or patterned bag can act as a statement piece. For example, a vibrant red bag can beautifully complement a black-and-white ensemble, adding a pop of color.

Functional Fashion:

Ensure your bag is both stylish and functional. Consider your daily needs—do you require a bag with multiple compartments, or is a sleek, minimalist design more your style? A structured handbag may convey professionalism, while a slouchy bag can give off a relaxed vibe.

Material and Texture:

The material of your bag plays a crucial role in its overall aesthetic and functionality. Leather bags often exude sophistication and durability, making them ideal for professional settings. Suede or canvas bags can lend a more casual, bohemian touch.

Consider mixing textures to create visual interest. A sleek leather bag paired with a soft knit scarf can create a balanced look that feels both polished and approachable.

Trend Awareness:

Stay informed about current trends but choose bags that reflect your personal style rather than simply following fleeting fashions. Classic styles, such as a structured tote or a crossbody bag, are timeless and can be invested in for long-term wear.

However, don't shy away from experimenting with trendy pieces. An on-trend mini bag or a quirky shape can be a fun addition to your collection and can refresh your outfits.

Practical Considerations:

Think about how you will use your bag. If you're often on the go, look for options that offer both style and practicality, such as bags with adjustable straps or those that can be worn in multiple ways.

Additionally, consider the weight of the bag itself. A lightweight bag can make a significant difference in your comfort, especially if you carry it for extended periods.

Incorporating jewelry, scarves, and bags into your outfits is not just about adding pieces; it's about creating a cohesive look that reflects your personal style. Each accessory has the potential to tell a story, to convey your mood, and to enhance your overall appearance.

As you explore the world of accessories, remember to:

Experiment: Don't be afraid to try new combinations. Mixing different styles and pieces can lead to unique and unexpected results that truly showcase your individuality.

Edit Your Choices: Sometimes, less is more. When in doubt, choose a few standout pieces rather than overwhelming your outfit with too many accessories. A well-chosen statement necklace or a beautifully patterned scarf can make a powerful impact.

Stay True to Yourself: Ultimately, the best accessories are those that resonate with you. Choose pieces that make you feel confident and comfortable, allowing you to express your unique identity.

By mastering the art of accessorizing with jewelry, scarves, and bags, you can elevate your style, ensuring that each outfit becomes a true reflection of who you are. Embrace the creativity of accessorizing and enjoy the transformation it brings to your wardrobe!

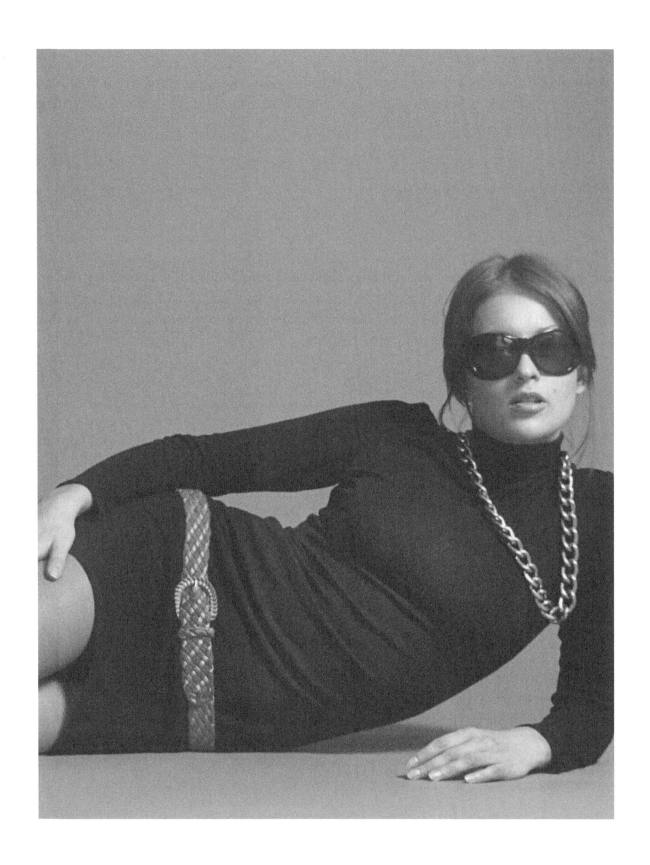

Adapting Accessories for Different Seasons

Accessorizing is not just about style; it's also about adapting to the changing seasons. Each season brings unique opportunities to refresh your look and incorporate accessories that enhance your outfits while providing comfort. Here's how to adapt your jewelry, scarves, and bags to suit the different seasons throughout the year.

Spring Accessories:

Spring is a time of renewal and freshness, making it ideal for vibrant colors and lightweight fabrics.

Jewelry:
Embrace floral and nature-inspired designs. Delicate earrings with pastel colors or floral motifs can add a touch of whimsy to your outfits.

Layering is key during this season, so consider mixing different metals and styles. A combination of gold and silver can create an interesting visual contrast.

Scarves:
Opt for lightweight scarves in bright colors or fun patterns. A lightweight cotton or silk scarf can be tied around your neck, used as a headband, or even wrapped around your wrist for a playful touch.

Floral prints or soft stripes can capture the essence of spring, adding a cheerful vibe to your look.

Bags:
Choose bags in light, airy materials like canvas or soft leather. Bright colors, such as pastel pinks or soft greens, can reflect the season's mood.

A crossbody bag or a small tote is perfect for outings, allowing you to keep your hands free while enjoying the blossoming outdoors.

Summer Accessories:

Summer is all about fun, relaxation, and vibrant colors. Accessories can enhance your breezy summer outfits.

Jewelry:
Lightweight, colorful jewelry is perfect for summer. Think beaded necklaces, shell bracelets, or stackable rings in bright hues.

Avoid heavy pieces that can feel uncomfortable in the heat; instead, opt for fun, playful designs that showcase your personality.

Scarves:
While summer scarves are often lighter, they can serve multiple purposes. Use a lightweight scarf as a head wrap to protect your hair from the sun or tie it around your bag for a splash of color.

Choose materials like chiffon or cotton that are breathable and comfortable in warmer temperatures.

Bags:
Summer bags should be functional yet stylish. Consider straw totes, beach bags, or colorful crossbody styles that can easily transition from day to night.

Bright colors and playful patterns are ideal, reflecting the carefree spirit of summer. Don't forget to choose a bag that can hold your essentials for beach days or picnics.

Fall Accessories

As the weather cools and leaves change, fall accessories can add warmth and depth to your outfits.

Jewelry:
Fall is the perfect time to incorporate richer, deeper colors into your jewelry. Think earthy tones like burgundy, forest green, or gold.

Layered pieces work well; consider wearing a cozy sweater with layered necklaces or statement earrings to add elegance to your autumn look.

Scarves:
Chunky knit scarves are a fall essential. They not only provide warmth but can also be used as a statement piece in your outfit.

Opt for plaid or autumnal colors like mustard, rust, and olive green. A large scarf can even double as a shawl on chilly evenings.

Bags:
Transition to bags made of thicker materials, such as leather or suede. Rich colors like deep brown, burgundy, or navy can enhance your fall wardrobe.

A structured handbag or a crossbody style can be both practical and chic for the season. Look for bags with autumn-inspired textures or embellishments.

Winter Accessories

Winter accessories are all about warmth, comfort, and festive flair.

Jewelry:

In winter, opt for statement pieces that stand out against heavier clothing. Think bold necklaces or oversized earrings that can shine through layers.

Consider incorporating metallics, such as silver or gold, which can add a touch of sparkle to your winter outfits.

Scarves:

Cozy, knitted scarves are essential for winter. Look for thicker materials that provide warmth and can be styled in various ways—wrapped, looped, or draped.

Darker hues or festive patterns can complement your winter wardrobe, adding both style and functionality.

Bags:

Choose bags that are both stylish and practical for winter weather. Waterproof materials can be beneficial in snowy or rainy conditions.

A larger bag with plenty of space for essentials, such as gloves, hats, and scarves, can keep you organized while looking chic. Opt for rich colors or textures, like a deep red leather bag, to embrace the season.

Adapting your accessories for different seasons is key to maintaining a fresh and stylish wardrobe year-round. By thoughtfully selecting pieces that complement the changing weather and trends, you can elevate your outfits and express your personal style in new ways.

In spring, opt for lighter fabrics and vibrant colors to reflect the blossoming nature around you. Think floral scarves, pastel handbags, and delicate jewelry that add a touch of freshness. As summer rolls in, embrace bold statements with oversized sunglasses, woven bags, and playful beach hats that not only protect you from the sun but also enhance your look.

When autumn arrives, transition to richer tones and textures. Chunky knit scarves, leather gloves, and stylish ankle boots can add warmth and sophistication to your ensemble. Finally, as winter sets in, don't shy away from luxurious accessories like

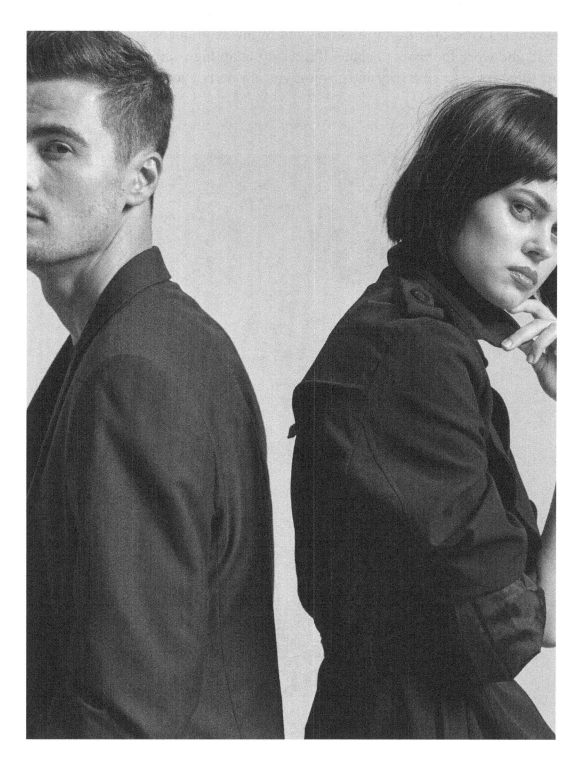

statement coats, cozy beanies, and elegant gloves that keep you warm while showcasing your fashion sense.

By rotating your accessories seasonally, you not only keep your wardrobe feeling new and exciting but also make the most of each season's unique offerings. This approach not only maximizes versatility but also allows you to invest in quality pieces that can be cherished and worn for years to come. Ultimately, adapting your accessories with the seasons enhances your creativity and ensures you always put your best foot forward, no matter the weather.

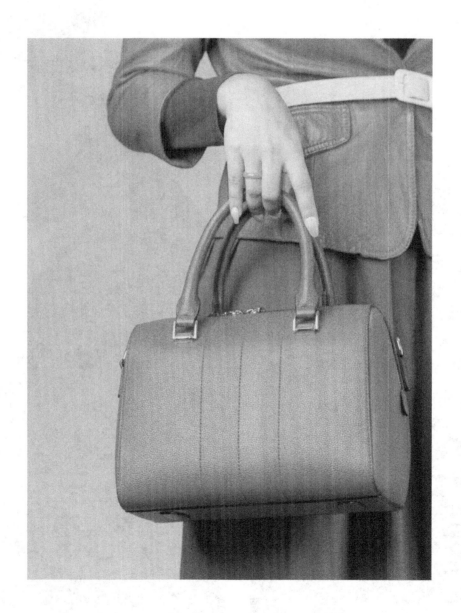

Chapter 7:

Shopping Smart

Thrift and Vintage Store Tips

Thrift and vintage stores are treasure troves for unique fashion finds, often filled with items that tell a story while offering style at a fraction of the retail price. Shopping in these stores can be both rewarding and economical, but it requires a bit of strategy. Here are some detailed tips to help you navigate thrift and vintage shopping like a pro.

Research Local Stores

Before embarking on your thrift shopping adventure, take the time to research thrift and vintage stores in your area. Look for reviews and recommendations online to identify those with a good reputation for quality merchandise. Use social media platforms or local community groups to find hidden gems. Some stores may specialize in certain types of clothing or eras, such as 80s retro or high-end designer pieces. Knowing what to expect can save you time and enhance your shopping experience.

Go in with an Open Mind

One of the joys of thrift shopping is the thrill of discovery. While it's helpful to have a general idea of what you're looking for—like a new jacket, a pair of jeans, or a statement accessory—be open to unexpected finds. You might stumble upon a vintage piece that perfectly complements your existing wardrobe or a unique accessory that adds flair to your outfits. The charm of thrift shopping lies in its unpredictability, so embrace the adventure!

Check for Quality

When shopping for secondhand items, it's important to inspect each piece carefully. Look for any signs of wear, such as fraying, stains, or broken zippers. Pay attention to the fabric quality; natural fibers like cotton, wool, and silk tend to hold up better over time than synthetic materials. Ensure that the item is structurally sound—check seams, buttons, and zippers. High-quality items can often be restored with a little care, so consider how much effort you're willing to invest in repairs.

Try Things On

Thrift and vintage stores can have varied sizing, so always try items on if possible. Sizing can differ significantly between brands and eras, and what looks good on the rack may not fit the same way on your body. Don't be discouraged if something doesn't fit perfectly; a skilled tailor can work wonders. Even if an item is slightly off, it might be worth purchasing if you can envision a simple alteration that will make it work for you.

Be Patient and Persistent

Finding the perfect piece in a thrift store can take time. Don't expect to find everything you need in one visit: it's often a process of trial and error. Make it a habit to check back regularly, as inventory changes frequently. Different stores have different cycles of donation and restocking, so what you didn't find last week might be there this week. Developing a relationship with your local thrift store can also yield benefits, such as insider knowledge of upcoming sales or new arrivals.

Understand Pricing

Familiarize yourself with the pricing structure of thrift and vintage stores. Some items may be priced higher due to their rarity, brand, or condition, while others might be incredibly affordable. Understanding what constitutes a fair price for vintage items can help you make informed purchasing decisions. Don't hesitate to negotiate prices in vintage stores where it's acceptable; a polite inquiry about pricing can sometimes lead to discounts.

Consider Upcycling

If you find an item that has potential but isn't quite right, consider upcycling it. Simple alterations, like shortening a dress, adding embellishments, or repurposing a piece into something new, can transform a thrifted item into something truly unique. This not only saves money but also allows you to express your creativity. There are countless online resources and tutorials available for DIY upcycling projects, making it easier than ever to breathe new life into your thrifted finds.

Shop with a Friend

Bringing a friend along can make thrift shopping a more enjoyable experience. They can offer a second opinion on items, help you stay within budget, and share in the thrill of the hunt. Plus, it's always fun to have someone to celebrate a great find with! You can also make a game out of it by challenging each other to find the best piece within a set budget, turning your shopping trip into a friendly competition.

Stay Organized

As you build your thrifted wardrobe, consider keeping an organized system for your finds. Create a dedicated space in your closet for thrifted items, and periodically assess your collection. This will help you avoid accumulating pieces you don't wear and encourage you to donate or sell items that no longer fit your style. An organized wardrobe not only makes it easier to get dressed but also allows you to appreciate the unique pieces you've curated over time.

Mind the Trends, But Stay True to Your Style

While thrift stores can be a great place to find trendy pieces, it's essential to stay true to your personal style. Trends come and go, but your unique style is what sets you apart. When browsing through thrift and vintage stores, focus on items that resonate with your personal aesthetic, rather than simply following the latest trends. An item might be trendy now, but if it doesn't reflect who you are, it may end up sitting in your closet unworn. Invest in pieces that make you feel confident and authentically you.

Learn About Vintage Fashion

Understanding the history of fashion can enrich your thrift shopping experience. Familiarize yourself with different fashion eras, key silhouettes, and iconic designers. This knowledge can help you spot valuable items and appreciate the craftsmanship that goes into vintage clothing. For example, knowing the difference between a true vintage piece from the 1960s and a modern reproduction can make a significant difference in both quality and value.

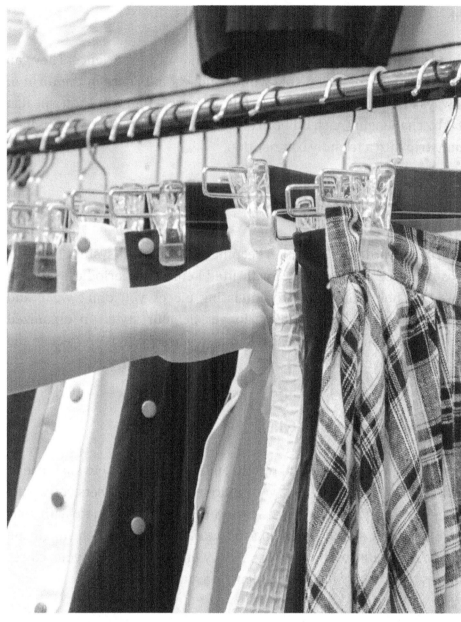

Visit Estate Sales and Flea Markets

Don't limit your thrift shopping to just secondhand stores. Estate sales and flea markets can offer incredible finds, often at lower prices than traditional thrift stores. At estate sales, you may discover high-quality vintage items or unique pieces that reflect a specific time period. Flea markets often host various vendors, giving you a wide range of styles and prices. Be prepared to negotiate, as many vendors expect some haggling.

Network with Other Thrift Shoppers

Join local thrift shopping groups or online forums where enthusiasts share tips, store recommendations, and styling ideas. Engaging with a community of like-minded individuals can elevate your thrift shopping experience. You might discover new stores, learn about upcoming sales, or even find friends to shop with. Sharing your thrifting victories and challenges can also motivate you to keep exploring.

Mind the Environment

Thrift shopping is not only a budget-friendly alternative; it's also an environmentally conscious choice. By choosing secondhand clothing, you contribute to reducing waste and promoting sustainability in the fashion industry. Take a moment to appreciate that each purchase is a step away from fast fashion and its detrimental impacts on the environment. This mindful approach can enhance your shopping experience, making it feel purposeful and rewarding.

Build a Capsule Wardrobe

As you curate your thrifted finds, consider building a capsule wardrobe—a collection of versatile pieces that can be mixed and matched to create various outfits. This approach not only simplifies your wardrobe but also emphasizes quality over quantity. By focusing on timeless essentials, you can create a cohesive style that transcends fleeting trends. Thrift stores are perfect for finding unique items that can serve as standout pieces in your capsule wardrobe.

Final Thoughts

Thrift and vintage shopping is not just about saving money; it's about embracing individuality, creativity, and sustainability in fashion. By following these tips, you can enhance your shopping experience and curate a wardrobe filled with unique, stylish pieces that reflect your personality. Remember, the goal is to enjoy the hunt and celebrate the stories behind each item you acquire. With patience, persistence, and a bit of creativity, you can transform your wardrobe into a collection of cherished finds that truly represent who you are. Happy thrifting!

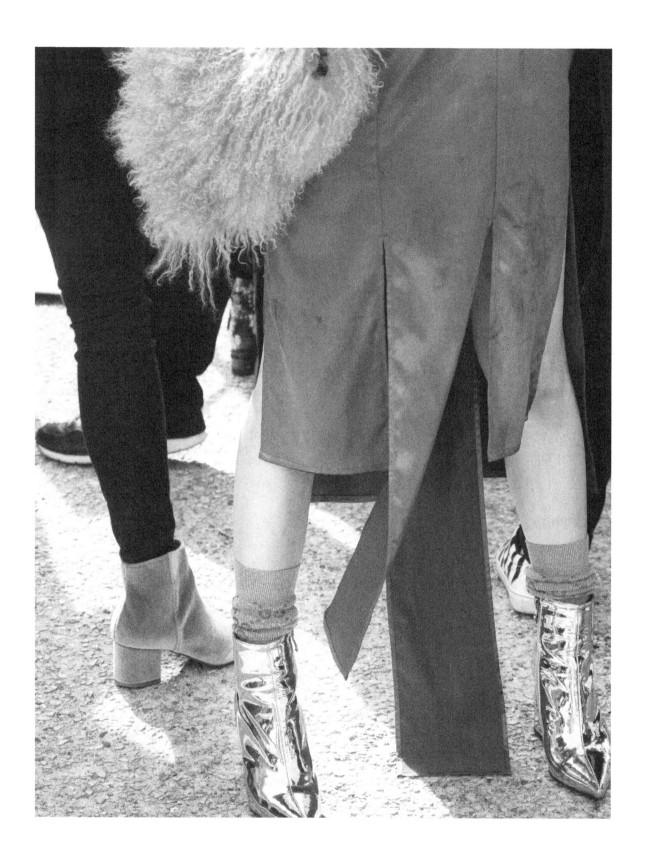

Embracing Sustainable and Ethical Fashion

In recent years, the fashion industry has witnessed a significant shift towards sustainability and ethical practices. As consumers become more aware of the environmental and social impacts of their purchases, embracing sustainable and ethical fashion has never been more important. This section will explore various aspects of sustainable fashion, providing insights and actionable tips for making responsible choices.

Understanding Sustainable Fashion

Eco-Friendly Materials:

Sustainable fashion starts with the materials used. Look for brands that prioritize eco-friendly fabrics such as organic cotton, linen, Tencel, and recycled polyester. These materials have a lower environmental impact compared to conventional fabrics, which often rely on harmful pesticides and extensive water usage.

Sustainable Production Processes:

Research brands that implement sustainable production practices. This includes reducing water consumption, minimizing waste through efficient manufacturing techniques, and using renewable energy sources. Brands that produce locally can also help reduce carbon emissions associated with transportation.

Supporting Ethical Brands

Researching Brand Ethics:

Invest time in learning about the brands you support. Look for certifications that indicate ethical practices, such as Fair Trade, GOTS (Global Organic Textile Standard), and B Corp. These certifications ensure that companies meet specific social and environmental standards.

Transparent Supply Chains:

Choose companies that are committed to transparency in their supply chains. Brands that share information about their sourcing, labor practices, and environmental impact allow consumers to make informed choices.

Buying Second-Hand

Thrift Shopping:

Explore local thrift stores, consignment shops, and online platforms for pre-loved clothing. This not only reduces waste but also promotes a circular economy where clothes are reused rather than discarded.

Clothing Swaps:

Organize or participate in clothing swaps with friends, family, or local community groups. These events allow you to refresh your wardrobe without spending money while promoting a sense of community and reducing textile waste.

Investing in Quality Over Quantity

Timeless Pieces:

Focus on purchasing high-quality, timeless garments that will last for years. Investing in classic pieces—like a well-fitted blazer, a little black dress, or sturdy jeans—can save money in the long run and reduce the need for frequent replacements.

Creating a Capsule Wardrobe:

Consider developing a capsule wardrobe composed of versatile pieces that can be mixed and matched. This minimalist approach encourages thoughtful purchasing and creates a cohesive wardrobe that can adapt to various occasions.

Mindful Shopping Habits

Limiting Impulse Buys:
Before making a purchase, ask yourself if you truly need the item and how it fits into your existing wardrobe. Implement a waiting period—such as 24 hours—before buying to help curb impulse purchases.

Caring for Your Clothes:
Proper care can significantly extend the life of your clothing. Follow washing instructions, avoid excessive drying, and store items appropriately to maintain their quality. Repairing garments instead of discarding them can also promote sustainability.

Educating Yourself and Others

Staying Informed:
Keep up with the latest trends and issues in sustainable fashion by following relevant blogs, podcasts, documentaries, and social media accounts dedicated to ethical fashion. Understanding the challenges and innovations in the industry can empower you to make better choices.

Spreading Awareness:
Share your knowledge with friends and family to encourage a collective shift towards more sustainable choices. Engaging in discussions about the impact of fast fashion can inspire others to rethink their shopping habits.

Advocating for Change

Supporting Policy Changes:
Get involved in initiatives that promote sustainable practices in the fashion industry. Advocate for legislation that supports ethical labor and environmental standards, and support organizations that work towards improving conditions in garment factories globally.

Challenging Brands:

Use social media platforms to hold brands accountable for their practices. Engage with companies by asking questions about their sustainability efforts and encouraging them to adopt more ethical methods. Consumer pressure can drive significant change in the industry.

Exploring Innovations in Sustainable Fashion

Technological Advancements:

Stay informed about innovations in sustainable fashion, such as biodegradable fabrics, 3D printing, and circular fashion initiatives. These technologies can reduce waste and improve the environmental impact of the fashion industry.

Sustainable Fashion Startups:

Support emerging brands that prioritize sustainability and ethical practices. Many startups are leading the way in innovative, eco-friendly designs, offering unique alternatives to traditional fashion.

Choosing Sustainable Accessories

Conscious Accessorizing:

Don't forget about accessories! Look for bags, shoes, and jewelry made from sustainable materials. Brands that focus on eco-friendly production can complement your sustainable wardrobe.

Upcycling and DIY:

Consider upcycling old accessories or creating your own. This not only saves money but also allows for personal expression and creativity. You can transform old jewelry, bags, or clothing into something new and unique.

Embracing Slow Fashion

Understanding Slow Fashion:

Slow fashion is the antithesis of fast fashion, emphasizing quality, craftsmanship, and sustainability. It encourages consumers to buy less and choose thoughtfully. By embracing slow fashion, you support artisans and local economies while reducing environmental impact.

Building Relationships with Brands:

Engage with brands that practice slow fashion. Cultivating a relationship with these companies allows you to learn more about their production processes and the stories behind their products, fostering a deeper connection to your purchases.

Exploring Rental and Subscription Services

Fashion Rentals:

Consider renting clothing for special occasions instead of buying new items that may only be worn once. Rental services offer a wide range of stylish options without the commitment of ownership, reducing waste in the fashion industry.

Subscription Services:

Explore subscription boxes that focus on sustainable and ethical fashion. These services often curate selections from conscious brands, allowing you to discover new styles while supporting sustainable practices.

Participating in Community Initiatives

Local Sustainability Projects:

Get involved in community initiatives focused on sustainability. This could include participating in local clothing drives, workshops on sustainable fashion, or events that promote awareness of environmental issues related to the fashion industry.

Advocacy and Education:

Partner with local organizations to advocate for sustainable practices within the community. Hosting educational workshops or discussions can raise awareness and inspire others to join the movement.

Reflecting on Your Fashion Identity

Personal Style:
Take time to reflect on your personal style and what sustainable fashion means to you. Understanding your fashion identity can guide your purchasing decisions and help you build a wardrobe that truly reflects who you are.

Emotional Connection:
Cultivating an emotional connection to your clothing can enhance your appreciation for sustainable fashion. By valuing the stories behind the pieces you own, you're more likely to care for them and make thoughtful choices in the future.

A Collective Movement Towards Change

Embracing sustainable and ethical fashion is not just a personal choice; it's a collective movement towards a more responsible and equitable industry. By making informed decisions, supporting ethical brands, and advocating for change, you contribute to a fashion landscape that prioritizes the well-being of both people and the planet.

Together, as conscious consumers, we can challenge the status quo and redefine the future of fashion. Every purchase is a vote for the kind of world we want to live in, and by choosing sustainability, we help shape an industry that aligns with our values. As you embark on your sustainable fashion journey, remember that small, consistent changes can lead to significant impacts. Happy shopping!

Chapter 8:

Expressing Yourself

Through Fashion

Understanding Fashion as a Form of Self-Expression

Fashion transcends mere fabric and stitching; it serves as a dynamic medium through which individuals communicate their identities, beliefs, and emotions. Each choice we make in our wardrobe is a brushstroke in the larger canvas of our lives, articulating our stories without the need for words. From the bold colors of a summer dress to the understated elegance of a tailored suit, every outfit conveys a message about who we are and how we wish to be perceived.

The Language of Fashion

Fashion operates as a complex language, rich with symbolism and meaning. Each garment we wear can signify different aspects of our lives, cultures, and personalities. For instance, donning a vintage band t-shirt might evoke a sense of nostalgia and a love for music, while a sharp, modern blazer may signal professionalism and ambition. The way we mix patterns, layer textures, and accessorize further enriches this dialogue, providing insight into our creativity, tastes, and values.

Accessories, often overlooked, also play a crucial role in self-expression. A statement necklace or a quirky pair of shoes can transform an outfit, adding layers of meaning that speak to our personalities. They can convey messages of rebellion, sophistication, or whimsy, making fashion a multi-dimensional form of expression.

Cultural Influences

Our fashion choices are deeply influenced by cultural backgrounds, societal norms, and the zeitgeist of the times. Different cultures celebrate unique styles, colors, and garments that carry profound historical significance. For example, traditional attire might reflect the values and customs of a particular community, while contemporary fashion may incorporate elements from various cultures, leading to a rich tapestry of global influences.

Embracing these cultural elements allows individuals to honor their heritage while simultaneously making a statement in modern contexts. Fashion can serve as a bridge connecting the past with the present, enabling us to showcase our roots while adapting to an ever-evolving landscape. In this way, global fashion trends can foster conversations about diversity and inclusivity, encouraging individuals to express their identities in ways that resonate with personal histories.

Emotional Expression

Fashion is intrinsically linked to our emotions and mental states. The choices we make in our attire often reflect how we feel on any given day. When we are confident, we may gravitate toward vibrant hues and bold patterns, while times of uncertainty may lead us to favor more subdued tones and comfortable silhouettes. The ability to dress according to our mood can be empowering, offering a sense of control and allowing us to navigate our feelings effectively.

This connection between fashion and emotion can be particularly therapeutic. For instance, a favorite outfit can evoke memories of joy and success, serving as a reminder of our strengths during challenging times. Conversely, experimenting with new styles can help us break free from emotional stagnation, encouraging personal growth and resilience. Understanding this relationship enables us to use fashion as a tool for emotional expression and self-care, fostering a deeper connection with ourselves.

Individuality vs. Conformity

While fashion provides a platform for self-expression, it can also present challenges regarding individuality and conformity. The pressure to adhere to trends or societal expectations can stifle creativity, making it difficult for individuals to express their true selves. However, true style emerges from authenticity. It is essential to recognize that fashion is not just about following the latest trends but about discovering what resonates with us personally and celebrating it.

The journey toward developing a personal style often involves experimentation and exploration. It requires us to step outside of our comfort zones and embrace our unique tastes, even if they diverge from mainstream fashion. By doing so, we cultivate a distinctive fashion identity that stands apart, allowing us to communicate our individuality boldly.

The Role of Fashion Icons and Influencers

Throughout history, fashion icons and influencers have played a significant role in shaping the way we perceive and express ourselves through clothing. Figures like Coco Chanel, Audrey Hepburn, and more contemporary influencers have redefined style norms, encouraging individuals to embrace their uniqueness. These icons often challenge societal standards, illustrating that fashion is not confined to a specific mold but is instead an evolving landscape that welcomes diverse interpretations.

Social media platforms have further amplified this phenomenon, allowing individuals to showcase their personal styles and connect with like-minded communities. The democratization of fashion through these platforms has made it possible for everyone to be an influencer in their own right, encouraging self-expression and creativity on a global scale.

In essence, fashion is a canvas upon which we paint our identities, a vibrant medium that allows us to showcase who we are, how we feel, and what we believe. By understanding fashion as a form of self-expression, we can make more conscious choices in our wardrobes that reflect our true selves.

As you curate your personal style, consider each outfit an opportunity to tell your story, to express your individuality, and to share your unique perspective with the world. Embrace the power of fashion not only as a means of adornment but as a profound form of communication that connects us to ourselves, to our cultures, and to each other.

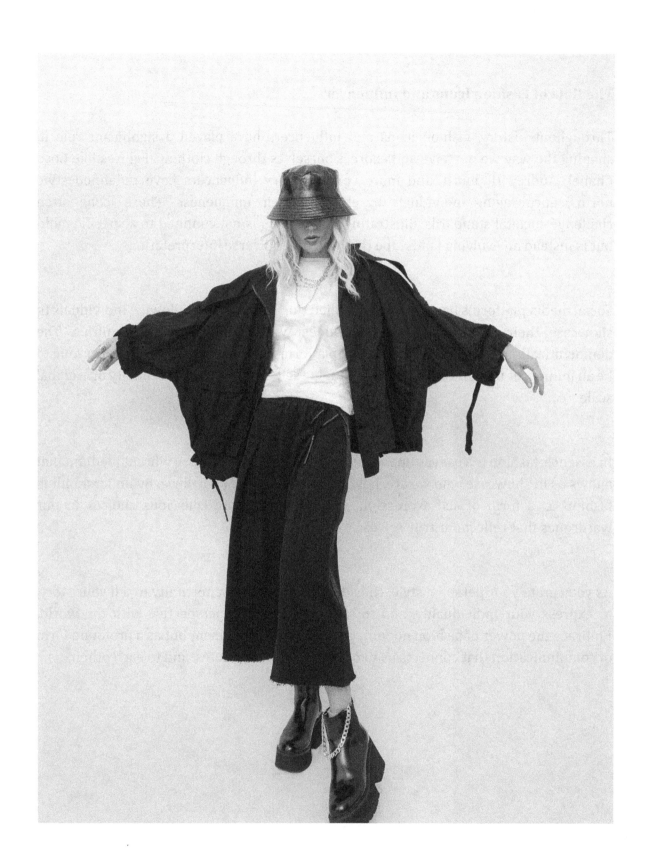

Trying New Styles with Confidence

Embracing new styles can be both exhilarating and intimidating. The prospect of stepping outside of our fashion comfort zones often brings a mix of excitement and anxiety. However, trying new styles is a vital part of personal expression and can significantly enhance our self-confidence. Here are some strategies to help you explore new looks with assurance.

Start Small

If the idea of a complete wardrobe overhaul feels overwhelming, begin with small changes. Introduce a single new item or accessory that reflects a different style. This could be a vibrant scarf, a unique piece of jewelry, or even a bold pair of shoes. These subtle additions can refresh your wardrobe and inspire you to explore further without feeling too drastic.

Experiment with Layers

Layering is an excellent way to experiment with various styles while maintaining comfort. By combining different textures, colors, and patterns, you can create unique outfits that reflect your personality. For example, try pairing a structured blazer over a casual graphic tee or layering a flowy dress with a denim jacket. This approach allows you to play with contrasts, making your outfits more dynamic and interesting.

Seek Inspiration

Inspiration can be found everywhere—from fashion magazines and social media platforms to street style and art. Follow fashion influencers who resonate with your aesthetic or explore hashtags that align with the styles you want to try. Creating a mood board or a digital collection of looks that inspire you can help you visualize your new style direction and motivate you to take the plunge.

Be Mindful of Fit

Regardless of the style you want to try, the fit of your clothing plays a crucial role in how confident you feel. Well-fitting clothes can enhance your silhouette and make you feel more comfortable in your skin. Don't hesitate to tailor pieces to achieve the perfect fit, as this can elevate any outfit and allow you to wear new styles with confidence.

Allow for Mistakes

Fashion is a journey of exploration, and not every attempt will yield the desired results. Embrace the possibility of making mistakes; they are part of the learning process. If an outfit doesn't feel right, take note of what didn't work and use that knowledge to refine your future choices. Remember, fashion is about personal expression, and it's okay to try and fail as you discover what truly resonates with you.

Celebrating Your Unique Journey

Every individual's fashion journey is unique, shaped by personal experiences, preferences, and cultural influences. Celebrate your individuality by recognizing that your style evolution is a reflection of your growth. Embrace the changes as you explore new trends and styles, and take pride in your journey of self-expression.

Fashion is a powerful tool for self-expression, allowing you to communicate your identity, emotions, and creativity. By trying new styles with confidence, you open yourself to a world of possibilities that can enhance your self-image and enrich your life. So go ahead, experiment, and let your wardrobe be a celebration of your unique journey.

Balancing Trends with Personal Preference

In the fast-paced world of fashion, trends come and go, often leaving individuals feeling pressured to keep up. However, while it's tempting to jump on every bandwagon, finding a balance between current trends and your personal preferences is key to developing a style that feels authentic and enduring. Here are some strategies to help you navigate this balance effectively.

Understanding Trends

Fashion trends are driven by a variety of factors, including cultural shifts, celebrity influence, and social media. While some trends are fleeting, others may have more lasting appeal. Understanding the context behind trends can help you discern which ones resonate with you and align with your personal style. Take the time to evaluate trends critically—ask yourself if they reflect your personality or if they are simply a passing fad.

Identify Your Signature Style

Establishing a signature style can serve as your anchor amidst the ever-changing landscape of fashion. Think about the elements that make you feel most confident and comfortable. This could include specific colors, patterns, or silhouettes that you consistently gravitate toward. By identifying these key components, you can integrate trendy pieces into your wardrobe while still staying true to your unique aesthetic.

Mix and Match

One of the most effective ways to balance trends with personal preference is to mix and match. Incorporate trendy items into outfits that reflect your established style. For example, if you love vintage-inspired clothing, try pairing a modern trend—like a popular print or color—with your favorite vintage pieces. This blending creates a fresh look that feels uniquely yours while still being relevant to current fashion.

Invest in Versatile Pieces

When exploring trends, consider investing in versatile pieces that can be styled in multiple ways. A trendy jacket, for instance, can be worn with various outfits, from casual to formal. This approach allows you to experiment with trends without overwhelming your wardrobe. Look for items that can transition across seasons and occasions, ensuring you get the most value out of your purchases.

Focus on Quality Over Quantity

In a world that often emphasizes fast fashion, prioritize quality over quantity when it comes to trendy items. Rather than accumulating numerous pieces that may only be relevant for a season, invest in well-made garments that you can wear for years to come. Quality items not only elevate your wardrobe but also allow you to express your style more authentically.

Stay True to Yourself

While it's easy to be swayed by popular opinion, remember to stay true to yourself. Fashion should be a reflection of who you are, not just what's trending. If a particular trend doesn't resonate with you, don't feel obligated to adopt it. Instead, focus on what makes you feel empowered and confident. Your style is a personal journey, and authenticity will always shine through.

Embrace Change and Growth

Your style will naturally evolve over time, influenced by personal experiences, changes in lifestyle, and shifts in interests. Embrace this growth as an opportunity to refine your fashion choices. Allow yourself to revisit trends you may have dismissed in the past or explore new styles that pique your interest.

Balancing trends with personal preference is essential for cultivating a wardrobe that feels both stylish and authentic. By understanding trends, identifying your signature style, and making thoughtful choices, you can navigate the fashion landscape with confidence.

Cultivating a Unique Fashion Identity

Cultivating a unique fashion identity involves understanding your personal style and using it as a canvas to express your individuality. To begin this journey, invest time in exploring what resonates with you. Your personal style is an extension of your personality and can be a reflection of your experiences, interests, and cultural background.

Start by looking through your wardrobe—what do you love to wear? Identify pieces that you always gravitate to, as well as those that make you feel confident and authentic. Ask yourself:

What colors do I gravitate towards? Colors can have a profound impact on mood and perception. Determine which hues uplift you and reflect your personality.

Which patterns or silhouettes make me feel comfortable? Consider whether you prefer structured clothing or flowy fabrics. This will help you curate a wardrobe that feels like "you."

Are there specific styles or trends that I admire but haven't tried yet? Don't shy away from experimentation. Fashion is about exploration, so allow yourself to step outside your comfort zone.

Keeping a style journal can be an invaluable tool in this process. Document outfits that inspire you, whether they come from social media, fashion magazines, or street style. Include notes about what you love about each look—this could be the color combination, the cut, or the overall vibe. Over time, patterns will emerge, showcasing your unique preferences and guiding your fashion choices.

As mentioned earlier, your fashion identity is not static; it evolves as you grow and change. Embrace versatility in your wardrobe by mixing and matching different styles. Experiment with different accessories, textures, and colors to see what combinations resonate most with you as you move along on your fashion journey.

And, as you cultivate your fashion identity, consider the impact of your choices on the environment and society. Aim to build a sustainable wardrobe by selecting quality pieces that align with your values. This might mean supporting ethical brands, exploring second-hand options, or investing in timeless pieces that will last for years.

Ultimately, the key to expressing yourself through fashion is confidence. Wear what makes you feel good, regardless of trends or societal expectations. When you feel good in what you wear, it radiates outward, influencing how others perceive you. Remember, fashion is a personal journey; there are no right or wrong choices.

To build confidence, practice positive self-talk and affirmations. Remind yourself that your style is valid and that expressing who you are through fashion is a beautiful form of art. Surround yourself with supportive friends who encourage your fashion endeavors, and don't hesitate to seek out inspiration from diverse sources.

Fashion is also deeply intertwined with culture and identity. Consider how your heritage, background, and personal experiences influence your style choices. Incorporating elements from your culture can create a rich and meaningful fashion identity. Whether it's traditional patterns, colors, or accessories, embracing your roots can foster a sense of pride and individuality. A good tip here is engaging with local artisans or designers who reflect your cultural background. Supporting these creators not only enhances your wardrobe but also celebrates diversity and creativity in fashion.

In summary, cultivating a unique fashion identity is a fulfilling endeavor that allows you to showcase your individuality. By exploring your style, embracing versatility, making conscious choices, and wearing your confidence, you create a fashion narrative that is distinctly yours. Your unique identity is waiting to be celebrated.

Chapter 9:

Maintaining and

Evolving Your Style

Wardrobe Organization and Maintenance

Maintaining a well-curated wardrobe is essential for expressing your personal style while ensuring practicality and ease of use. An organized closet not only saves time during your daily routine but also helps you appreciate your clothing choices more fully. Here are some effective strategies for wardrobe organization and maintenance that will keep your style fresh and relevant.

Declutter Regularly

Start with a thorough review of your wardrobe. Set aside time every season to assess what you truly wear and love. Items that haven't been worn in the past year should be considered for donation or resale. This process not only creates space but also allows you to focus on pieces that resonate with your current style.

Categorize Your Clothing

Organizing your wardrobe by category—such as tops, bottoms, dresses, and outerwear—can significantly enhance visibility and accessibility. Within each category, consider further organizing by color, season, or occasion. This structured approach makes it easier to mix and match outfits, ensuring you maximize the potential of every piece.

Invest in Quality Hangers and Storage Solutions

The right hangers can help maintain the shape of your garments. Opt for padded hangers for delicate items, wooden ones for heavy coats, and non-slip options for slippery fabrics. For folded items, consider storage bins or shelves that keep your clothes visible and accessible. Proper storage prevents wear and tear, prolonging the life of your favorite pieces.

Care for Your Clothes

Understanding how to properly care for your clothing is essential for maintenance. Follow washing instructions meticulously and invest in a good quality detergent. Regularly check for loose threads, missing buttons, or signs of wear, and address these issues promptly. This proactive approach will help keep your wardrobe looking its best.

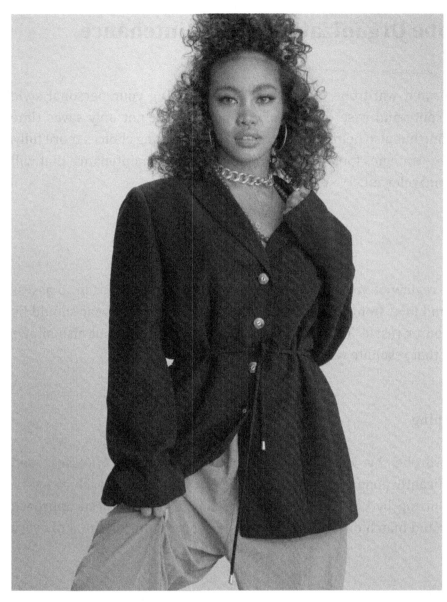

Adapt to Changing Trends and Personal Growth

As your personal style evolves, so should your wardrobe. Stay attuned to current fashion trends, but also reflect on your personal growth. If certain pieces no longer align with your identity or lifestyle, consider letting them go. Embrace new styles gradually by adding a few trendy items each season, which can refresh your look without overwhelming your existing wardrobe.

Create a Seasonal Transition Plan

As seasons change, so too should your wardrobe. Develop a plan for transitioning your clothing: rotate seasonal items in and out of your main wardrobe space. Consider storing off-season clothes in bins to free up space for current season essentials. This not only keeps your closet tidy but also allows you to rediscover pieces you may have forgotten.

Document Your Outfits

Keeping a visual record of your outfits can be incredibly beneficial. Consider taking photos of your looks to help you remember combinations that work well. This can also serve as inspiration for future outfits, making it easier to pull together stylish ensembles quickly.

Be Open to Experimentation

Finally, maintaining and evolving your style is an ongoing journey. Don't be afraid to experiment with new looks and combinations. Attend local fashion events, browse online platforms, or engage with style communities for fresh ideas. Your wardrobe should reflect who you are now, and that may change over time.

By implementing these strategies, you can maintain a wardrobe that not only embodies your style but also adapts to your evolving tastes and lifestyle. Embrace the process of organizing and caring for your clothing as a key part of your personal style journey—one that allows you to express your individuality creatively and confidently.

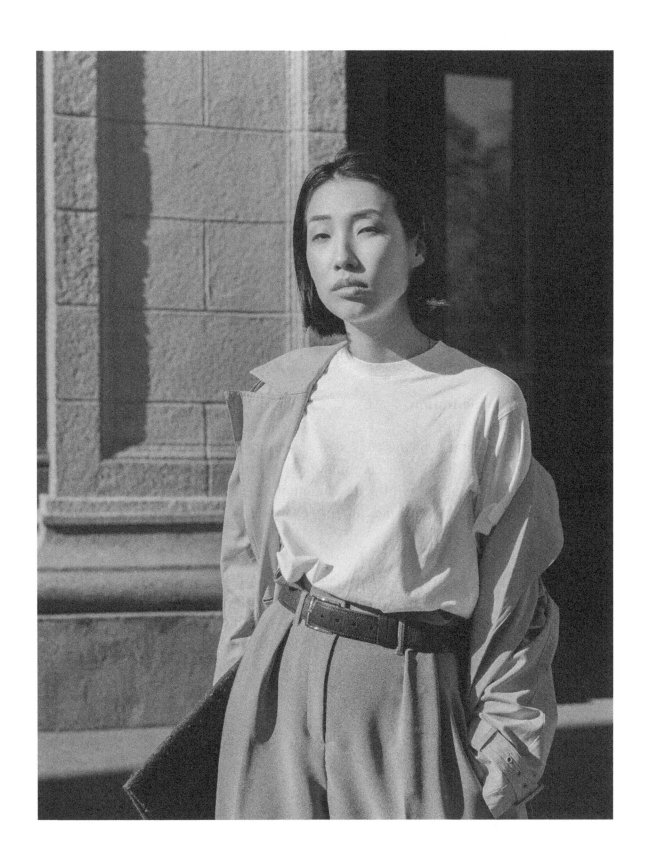

Updating Your Style with Life Changes

Life is a series of transitions, and each phase often brings shifts in our personal style. Whether it's a new job, a significant move, or changes in your personal relationships, having children, adapting your wardrobe to reflect these life changes can be empowering. Here are several ways to update your style in response to evolving circumstances:

Assess Your New Environment

When you experience a major life change, take time to evaluate your new surroundings. A move to a different climate or city can drastically influence your clothing needs. For instance, relocating to a warmer climate might mean investing in lighter fabrics and more casual styles, while a new job in a corporate setting may require a more polished wardrobe. Consider what works best for your new environment and adjust accordingly.

Reflect on Your Current Roles

As your responsibilities change—whether due to a new job, parenthood, or other commitments—your wardrobe should reflect these new roles. Think about the activities you'll be engaged in and the impression you want to convey. Incorporate versatile pieces that can transition from professional settings to casual outings, ensuring you feel confident in all aspects of your life.

Identify and Embrace New Inspirations

Life changes often lead to new interests or perspectives. Use this opportunity to explore different styles or aesthetics that resonate with your current self. Follow fashion influencers, browse magazines, or explore social media platforms for fresh ideas. Don't hesitate to experiment with new colors, patterns, or silhouettes that align with your evolving identity.

Purge and Refresh Your Wardrobe

With each life change, take the opportunity to re-evaluate your wardrobe. Remove items that no longer serve you or reflect who you are. This process of purging can be liberating and paves the way for introducing new pieces that better align with your current lifestyle. Consider donating or selling clothes to make space for fresh additions that inspire you.

Invest in Key Pieces

As your style evolves, identify a few key pieces that can enhance your wardrobe. This could be a tailored blazer for work, a stylish pair of shoes, or a statement accessory that adds flair to your outfits. Prioritize quality over quantity and choose items that will stand the test of time, ensuring they remain relevant as your style continues to develop.

Incorporate Seasonal Updates

Life changes often coincide with the changing seasons. Use this time to refresh your wardrobe accordingly. As seasons shift, invest in new pieces that reflect the weather and activities you'll be participating in. Seasonal updates not only keep your wardrobe functional but also allow you to experiment with new trends that align with your evolving style.

Seek Feedback and Support

Sometimes, a fresh perspective can help you navigate style changes. Don't hesitate to seek feedback from friends or family whose opinions you trust. They may offer insights that you hadn't considered, helping you refine your style choices. Additionally, consider engaging with a stylist or fashion consultant for personalized advice tailored to your new lifestyle.

Embrace the Journey

Updating your style is a continual process, and it's important to embrace the journey. Allow yourself the freedom to make mistakes and discover what truly resonates with you. Every phase of life is an opportunity for growth, and your wardrobe should reflect your unique journey. Celebrate the changes and enjoy the process of evolving your style in tandem with your life.

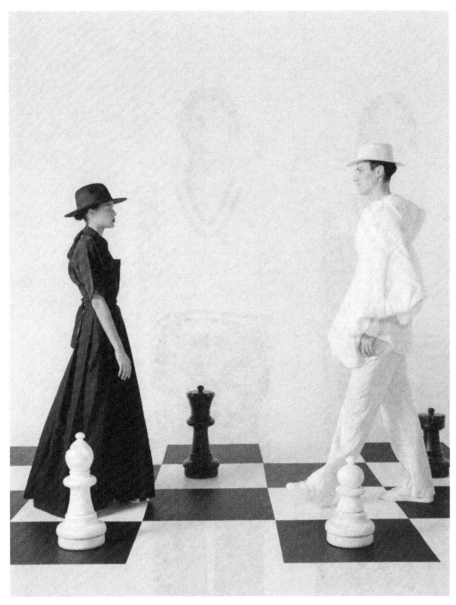

As you can see, by updating your wardrobe in response to life changes, you not only enhance your personal style but also cultivate a sense of confidence and authenticity. Your clothing is a powerful expression of who you are, and as you navigate the various chapters of life, let your wardrobe evolve alongside you.

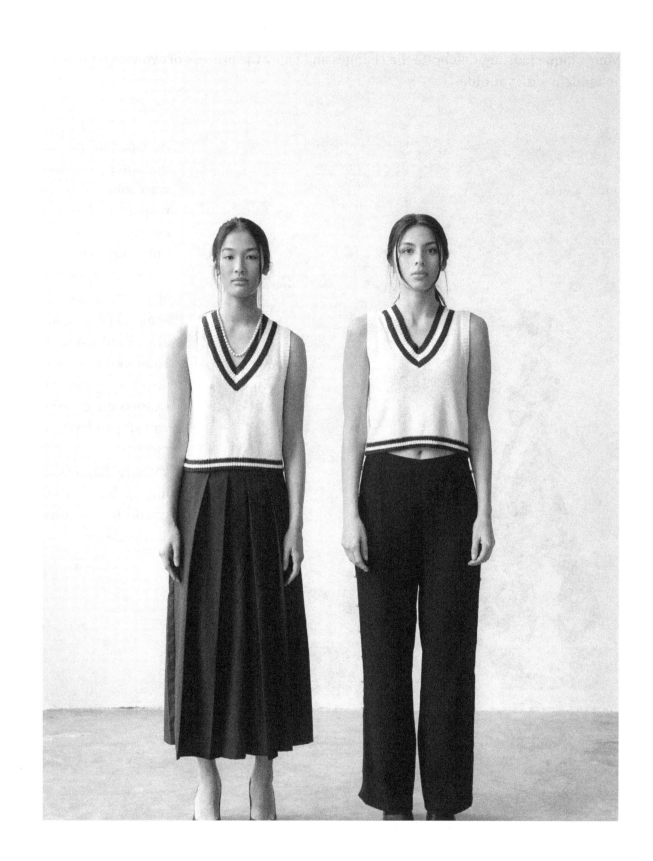

Staying Inspired in Fashion

Fashion is one of these things that is ever evolving, and staying inspired is key to maintaining a dynamic and personalized style. Whether you're looking for fresh ideas to revamp your wardrobe or simply want to keep your fashion sense vibrant, here are some effective strategies to keep your creativity flowing.

Follow Fashion Influencers and Creators

Social media platforms like Instagram, TikTok, and Pinterest are treasure troves of fashion inspiration. Follow influencers whose styles resonate with you and explore diverse aesthetics. This exposure can introduce you to new trends, styling techniques, and outfit combinations that you might not have considered before. Just remember to curate your feed to reflect styles that genuinely inspire you.

Explore Fashion Blogs and Magazines

Fashion blogs and magazines can provide in-depth insights into upcoming trends, styling tips, and interviews with designers. Regularly reading these resources can help you stay updated on the latest in the fashion world while offering ideas that align with your personal taste. Look for publications that celebrate diverse styles and perspectives to broaden your fashion horizons.

Visit Local Boutiques and Thrift Stores

Exploring local boutiques and thrift stores can be a fun way to discover unique pieces that resonate with your style. These shops often carry items that aren't found in mainstream retail, allowing you to curate a wardrobe that feels truly one-of-a-kind. Take your time browsing, and don't hesitate to try on pieces that catch your eye—even if they're outside your usual style.

Attend Fashion Events and Shows

If possible, attend fashion shows, trunk shows, or local fashion events. These experiences can provide firsthand insight into upcoming trends and allow you to see how styles are presented on the runway. Engaging with fellow fashion enthusiasts can also spark new ideas and discussions about personal style.

Experiment with DIY Projects

Get creative by incorporating DIY projects into your fashion routine. Upcycling old garments or customizing pieces can give new life to your wardrobe while allowing you to express your individuality. Whether it's adding embellishments, dyeing fabrics, or altering silhouettes, DIY fashion can be a fulfilling way to stay inspired.

Keep a Style Journal

Maintaining a style journal can be a powerful tool for self-reflection and inspiration. Document your outfits, jot down ideas, and collect images or swatches that inspire you. By keeping track of what you love, you can identify patterns in your style and continually refine your wardrobe choices.

Engage with Fashion Communities

Join online or local fashion communities where you can share ideas, ask for advice, and exchange inspiration with like-minded individuals. Platforms like Reddit, Facebook groups, or local meet-up events can provide a supportive space to discuss trends, seek feedback, and find encouragement in your style journey.

Travel and Experience New Cultures

Traveling can profoundly impact your fashion perspective. Experiencing new cultures and their unique styles can inspire you to incorporate different elements into your wardrobe. Whether it's the colors, fabrics, or silhouettes you encounter, travel can open your eyes to fresh ideas and trends that resonate with your personal aesthetic.

Stay Open to Change

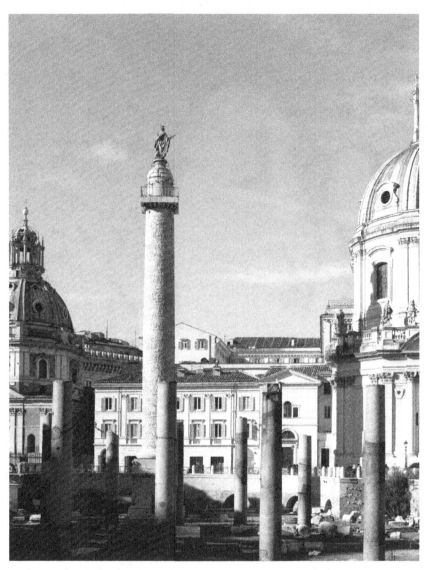

Lastly, remember that fashion is about experimentation and evolution. Allow yourself to be open to change and new ideas. Your style should reflect who you are at any given moment, and it's okay to try out different looks until you find what truly resonates with you. Embrace the journey and enjoy the process of discovering what inspires you.

By actively seeking inspiration and remaining engaged with the fashion world, you can keep your style fresh and exciting. Fashion is a form of self-expression, and the more you explore and experiment, the more you'll discover about your own unique aesthetic. Embrace the inspiration around you, and let it guide you as you curate a wardrobe that reflects your ever-evolving self.

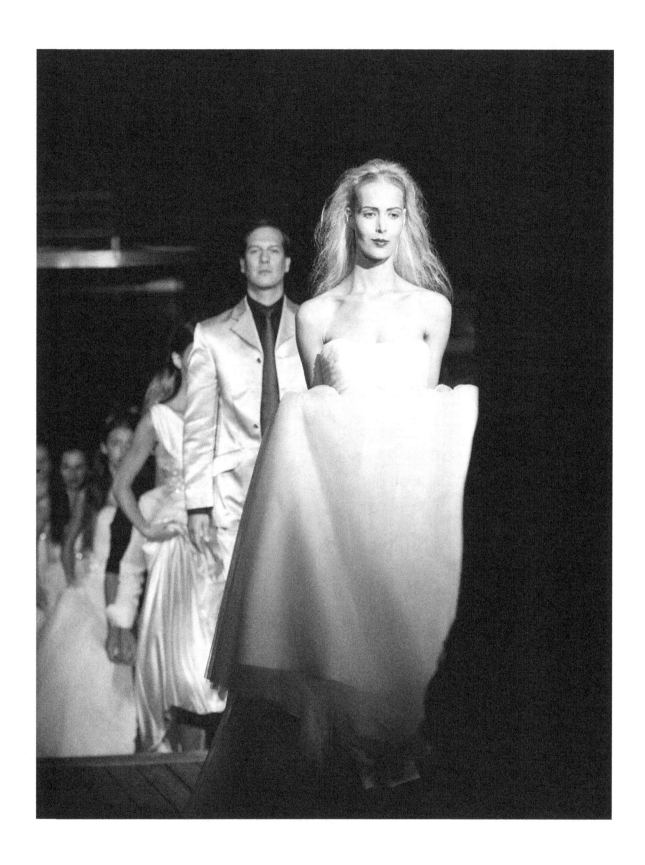

Embracing Style Evolution and Growth

Embracing the evolution of your style can be a liberating and empowering journey and this is what we will cover in this section. Below are some key principles to help you navigate this process and celebrate your unique fashion evolution.

Acknowledge Your Journey

Recognizing where you started and how far you've come is crucial. Take time to reflect on your past style choices and the reasons behind them. Whether you've embraced a more sophisticated look, adopted a minimalist approach, or explored bold colors and patterns, each phase has contributed to your current identity. Celebrate these changes as milestones in your personal fashion journey.

Stay True to Yourself

As your style evolves, it's essential to remain authentic. While trends can be tempting, ensure that your wardrobe reflects your true self. Resist the urge to conform to external pressures; instead, curate pieces that resonate with your values, lifestyle, and personality. When you dress in a way that feels genuine, you'll exude confidence and comfort, making a lasting impression.

Experiment Without Fear

As mentioned earlier in this book, don't be afraid to step outside your comfort zone and try new styles, colors, and silhouettes. Whether it's a daring accessory or an unexpected outfit combination, allow yourself the freedom to explore. Even if certain styles don't work out, each attempt is a valuable step in understanding your preferences and refining your aesthetic.

Learn from Mistakes

Mistakes are a natural part of the style evolution process. Instead of viewing them as failures, see them as learning opportunities. Analyze what didn't work and use that knowledge to make better choices in the future. This mindset will not only help you grow but also instill resilience and adaptability in your fashion journey.

Curate a Signature Look

As you evolve, consider developing a signature look that encapsulates your style. This could include a specific color palette, a favorite accessory, or a go-to outfit formula. A signature style can serve as a foundation that you build upon, allowing you to explore new trends while maintaining a cohesive aesthetic that feels uniquely you.

Be Open to Feedback

Engaging with friends, family, or fashion communities can provide valuable insights into your evolving style. Be open to constructive feedback and use it to refine your choices. Sometimes, an outside perspective can highlight aspects of your style that you may not have considered, helping you grow in ways you hadn't anticipated.

Celebrate Milestones

Recognize and celebrate your style milestones, whether it's mastering a new look or successfully incorporating a trend into your wardrobe. Documenting these moments in a style journal or sharing them on social media can reinforce your progress and inspire others on their own journeys. Celebrating achievements fosters a positive relationship with your evolving style.

Embrace Change as a Constant

Understanding that change is a constant in life will help you embrace your style evolution more readily. Your fashion choices will naturally shift as you grow and experience new phases in your life. Instead of resisting these changes, welcome them as part of your ongoing journey. Each new chapter brings opportunities for reinvention and self-discovery.

Find Inspiration in Diversity

Seek inspiration from various sources, including different cultures, art forms, and historical styles. Embracing diversity in fashion can open your eyes to new ideas and perspectives, enriching your personal style. Incorporating elements from various influences can create a unique blend that reflects your individuality and experiences.

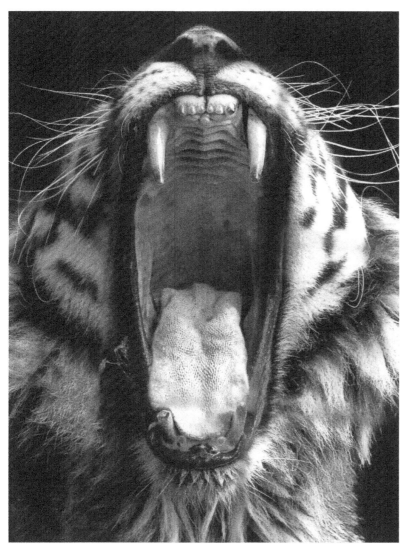

Practice Self-Compassion

Finally, be kind to yourself throughout your style evolution. It's normal to have moments of uncertainty or to feel disconnected from your current wardrobe. Allow yourself grace during these times, and remember that fashion is a journey, not a destination. Embracing self-compassion will empower you to explore your style without fear or judgment.

By embracing style evolution and growth, you will notice that this journey is about more than just clothing; it's about expressing your identity and celebrating your unique path. Allow your style to evolve as you do and enjoy the process of discovering the many facets of your fashion narrative.

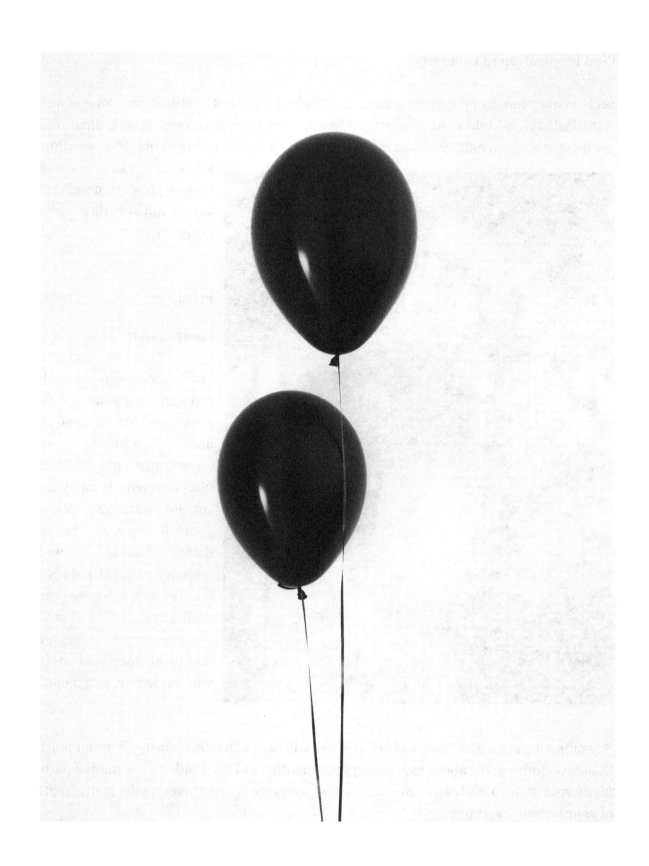

Conclusion

Key Takeaways and Encouragement

We hope you have enjoyed this book, "Know Your Fashion: Uncovering and Expressing Your Clothing Style." As you reflect on the insights and tips shared within these pages, we encourage you to embrace your unique style journey. Here are some key takeaways from the book and further inspiration to keep you motivated throughout this journey:

Discover Your Unique Style:

Take the time to explore your personal preferences, lifestyle, and inspirations to uncover a style that resonates authentically with you. Embrace the journey of self-discovery through fashion, allowing your clothing choices to reflect your individuality and personality. Celebrate what makes you feel confident, empowered, and true to yourself in every outfit you wear.

Build a Versatile Wardrobe:

Focus on curating a versatile and functional wardrobe that aligns with your personal style. Invest in essential pieces that can be mixed and matched to create various outfits suitable for different occasions. By blending basics with statement pieces, you can express your creativity, adapt to changing trends, and showcase your unique fashion identity confidently.

Embrace Self-Expression:

Use fashion as a powerful form of self-expression, allowing you to communicate your personality, values, and emotions through your clothing choices. Be bold, experiment with different styles, and express yourself authentically without fear or hesitation. Your wardrobe is a reflection of your inner self; let it be a source of empowerment and joy in showcasing who you are to the world.

Stay Informed About Trends:

Navigate the dynamic world of fashion by staying informed about trends while staying true to your personal style. Distinguish between fleeting fads and timeless pieces that resonate with you. Make informed fashion choices that reflect your preferences, values, and individuality, allowing you to incorporate trends in a way that feels genuine and authentic to you.

Overcome Fashion Challenges:

Acknowledge and address any challenges you may face in the realm of fashion, whether related to body image, inspiration, or uncertainty about your style preferences. Seek practical solutions, encouragement, and support to overcome these obstacles, embracing your uniqueness and individuality in the process. Remember, fashion should be a source of empowerment and confidence, not a source of stress or self-doubt.

Cultivate Confidence:

Cultivate a sense of confidence in your clothing choices by embracing your body, celebrating your uniqueness, and fostering self-love and acceptance. Wear outfits that make you feel comfortable, confident, and empowered. We encourage you to embrace your individuality, express yourself boldly, and radiate confidence in every fashion decision you make. Trust in your instincts, embrace your style evolution, and let your wardrobe be a reflection of your beautiful and authentic self.

Finally, embrace the journey of self-discovery through fashion with enthusiasm, curiosity, and self-assurance. Use your clothing as a canvas to express your personality, creativity, and inner essence to the world. The process of exploring different looks, experimenting with new styles, and evolving your personal fashion identity can be a very enjoyable one, knowing that your wardrobe speaks volumes about the remarkable person you are.

And if you enjoyed this book, don't hesitate to leave us a review at the place of purchase, and don't hesitate to visit our website at alloflare.com.

A Letter from the Author

Dear Readers,

I want to take a moment to express my heartfelt gratitude to each of you. I hope you find inspiration and empowerment within these pages as you embark on your journey of self-discovery and unique style. Fashion is more than just clothing; it's a powerful form of self-expression that allows us to communicate our identities to the world. In a society that often emphasizes conformity, embracing individuality in fashion is an act of courage and creativity.

As I reflect on this journey, I encourage you to explore your personal style, experiment with colors, textures, and silhouettes that resonate with who you truly are. This journey isn't just about aesthetics; it's about building confidence, empowerment, and authenticity. When you wear what feels right, you project an energy that is magnetic and inspiring, inviting others to embrace their uniqueness.

I've seen the fashion industry begin to recognize the importance of diversity and representation. Designers are increasingly creating collections that celebrate a wide range of body types, ethnicities, and cultural backgrounds. This shift is crucial because it allows individuals from all walks of life to see themselves reflected in fashion, enriching the industry with new voices and stories. Think about the impact of streetwear, rooted in subcultures that challenge mainstream aesthetics. By wearing pieces that honor these origins, you celebrate your individuality while paying homage to the rich history behind these styles.

As we navigate this journey, let's remember the importance of self-acceptance. By celebrating both our uniqueness and shared similarities, we can elevate our style into something truly extraordinary. Embrace what sets you apart while recognizing our common threads to create a personal expression that is uniquely yours. By doing so, we enrich our lives and create a more colorful, inclusive, and inspiring world for everyone.

Thank you from the bottom of my heart for being part of this journey. Your support has made "Know Your Fashion: Uncover and Express Your Clothing Style" a reality, and I am forever grateful for each of you.

With all my best,

Ally G.

Made in the USA
Monee, IL
29 January 2025

11247035R00109